Somatic Exercises: The Essential Guide to a Regulated Nervous System

50+ Effective Techniques to Soothe Stress and Anxiety, Release Trauma, and Activate the Power of the Vagus Nerve in Under 7 Minutes a Day

Ashlyn Summers

© Copyright 2024 - All rights reserved.

The content contained within this book may not be reproduced, duplicated or transmitted without direct written permission from the author or the publisher.

Under no circumstances will any blame or legal responsibility be held against the publisher, or author, for any damages, reparation, or monetary loss due to the information contained within this book, either directly or indirectly.

Legal Notice:

This book is copyright protected. It is only for personal use. You cannot amend, distribute, sell, use, quote or paraphrase any part, or the content within this book, without the consent of the author or publisher.

Disclaimer Notice:

Please note the information contained within this document is for educational and entertainment purposes only. All effort has been executed to present accurate, up to date, reliable, complete information. No warranties of any kind are declared or implied. Readers acknowledge that the author is not engaged in the rendering of legal, financial, medical or professional advice. The content within this book has been derived from various sources. Please consult a licensed professional before attempting any techniques outlined in this book.

By reading this document, the reader agrees that under no circumstances is the author responsible for any losses, direct or indirect, that are incurred as a result of the use of the information contained within this document, including, but not limited to, errors, omissions, or inaccuracies.

Table of Contents

INTRODUCTION	5
PART 1: THE FOUNDATIONAL PILLARS	9
THE PRINCIPLES OF SOMATIC THERAPY	11
Definition of Somatic Therapy	11
Benefits of Somatic Therapy	14
Three Methods in Somatic Experiencing	16
Things You Should Know	17
PART 2: SOMATIC EXERCISES	19
BODY AWARENESS	21
Exercise 1: Body Scan	22
Exercise 2: Understanding Misuse vs. Proper Use	24
Exercise 3: Lessening Effort	27
Exercise 4: Lying-Down Work	29
Exercise 5: Monkey Stance	31
Exercise 6: Supportive Touch	34
GROUNDING	37
Exercise 7: Squeeze Hug	38
Exercise 8: Tuning Into the Senses	40
Exercise 9: Standing in Your Power	42
Exercise 10: Tree Grounding Visualization	44
Exercise 11: Slight Chest Compressions	46
Exercise 12: Protective Force Fields	48
BREATHWORK	51
Exercise 13: Voo Breathing	52
Exercise 14: 4–5–6 Breathing	54
Exercise 15: Pursed-Lip Breathing	56
Exercise 16: Diaphragmatic Breathing	58
Exercise 17: Double Inhale Technique	61
Exercise 18: Three-Dimensional Breathing	63
Exercise 19: Whispered "Ah" (Rediscovering Your Voice)	66
MOVEMENT THERAPY	71
Exercise 20: Bilateral Stimulation	72
Exercise 21: Brain Tapping	76
Exercise 22: Snap–Snap–Clap Rhythm	78
Exercise 23: Emotional Freedom Technique (EFT)	80
Exercise 24: Body Tapping (Qigong)	83
Exercise 25: Eye Movement Routine (Qigong)	86
Exercise 26: Swaying Bamboo (Qigong)	88
Exercise 27: Shaking (Qigong)	90
Exercise 28: Opening (Qigong)	93
Exercise 29: Lifting the Ball (Qigong)	95
Exercise 30: Frolicking in Water (Qigong)	97

    Exercise 31: Lizard Walk 100

RELEASING TENSION **103**
    Exercise 32: Softening the Gaze 104
    Exercise 33: Cupping the Eyes 106
    Exercise 34: Release Neck and Shoulder Tension 108
    Exercise 35: Retraining the Neck and Shoulders 110
    Exercise 36: Progressive Muscle Relaxation 112
    Exercise 37: Release Psoas 114
    Exercise 38: Release Stomach Tension 118
    Exercise 39: Psoas Pandiculation 120

ACTIVATING THE VAGUS NERVE **125**
    Exercise 40: Ear Pull 126
    Exercise 41: Salamander Exercise 128
    Exercise 42: Vagus Nerve Activation Routine 130
    Exercise 43: Polyvagal Vagus Nerve Reset 134
    Exercise 44: Butterfly Hug 136
    Exercise 45: Hand Reflexology 138
    Exercise 46: Humming 142
    Exercise 47: Gargling 144

EMOTIONAL EXPRESSION AND RELEASE **147**
    Exercise 48: Twist and Growl 148
    Exercise 49: Laughter Yoga 150
    Exercise 50: Wiping the Table 152
    Exercise 51: Ecstatic Dancing 154

PART 3: 28-DAY PLAN **157**

CONCLUSION **159**

REFERENCES **163**

BONUSES: Video Exercises + 28-Day Plan Tracker for Free!

Ready for your **FREE** videos with **LIFETIME** access? 🎥

Want to get early access to my future books for **FREE**? 📚

Scan the QR code with your mobile or tablet below and tell us where to send your gifts!

OR

Visit this link:

subscribepage.io/j5p4gI

Congrats on embarking on your somatic journey!

My deepest gratitude goes to my teachers, mentors, and loved ones who have been part of this amazing journey. Your wisdom, encouragement, and boundless generosity have been instrumental in bringing this book to life. It's a true privilege and an honor to share this powerful work with readers seeking to transform their lives. This book is as much yours as it is mine.

With Gratitude,
Ashlyn

Introduction

Have you ever seen a child struggling with a backpack that's loaded with textbooks? It can be a struggle to lug all that weight around. I remember being a student and what it felt like to drop all that weight at the end of the day. There would be a few moments when I felt almost weightless with relief.

Living with unresolved trauma is like carrying that overweight backpack but never being able to put it down. It can make even small tasks seem insurmountable, and it impacts every part of your everyday life. And it's a more prevalent issue than you might realize. Recent studies have shown that 70% of the global population will experience a potentially traumatic moment at least once in their lives (World Health Organization, 2024).

When we don't process and release trauma, we look a bit like that student with the massive backpack, legs shaking as they walk to school. We're weighed down, exhausted, and sometimes even in pain.

Trauma is not a singular moment or even a series of moments. Trauma is what sticks around long after the painful event. Just because you've left behind the toxic environment, the abuse, the accident—whatever caused the trauma—it doesn't mean you aren't still living with the lasting effects.

It can feel lonely and a little scary to acknowledge your trauma, but just know that you aren't alone in those feelings. I've been at the beginning of this journey and, let me tell you, it has been nothing short of extraordinary.

When I was in my 20s, I suffered from intense anxiety, stress, and depression. Every day felt overwhelming, and there were times when it felt like too much just to get out of bed. There were other times I'd binge eat. Anything to escape the feelings inside my own body. Then, the next day, I would starve myself and work out to the point of exhaustion, out of shame for what I'd done the night before. I even found myself overindulging in alcohol. I was trying so desperately to escape, but everything just furthered the spiral.

It was a friend who recommended that I see a somatic therapist. At that point, I was desperate for anything that might work. So, I gave it a shot. When I went, I began to realize how unsafe I felt in my body. Through the tools and techniques I learned, I began to feel safer in my body. Before too long, I realized I wasn't trying to disconnect or dissociate anymore. Instead, my body was a sanctuary that I respected and lived in tune with. That emotional weight that I had been unknowingly carrying like a backpack full of textbooks—it started to lift. Sometimes, it would be subtle, and other times, immense. But I could feel the progress.

So, what *is* somatic therapy? To give you an idea, here's a fun fact: The word *somatic* comes from a Greek root meaning "body." This form of therapy seeks to bring the psychological and physical together to heal the whole person. Trauma isn't just stored in the mind, after all. It is also stored in the body.

Somatic therapy takes a dual approach to healing, focusing not just on thoughts but also on how emotions are felt physically. It goes beyond talk therapy, instead helping you feel safe in your body, fully feeling what you need to feel.

Because there *is* a connection between mind and body. This knowledge isn't new. It was understood by ancient traditions, long before modern therapy was developed. This intimate connection between the mind and the body is often the "missing piece" that helps individuals on their path of healing.

It goes both ways, too! Modern studies have found that stress and trauma can manifest in physical symptoms. This could look like tension headaches, or even chronic pain. That's not to say it's "all in your head." The pain is very real. But the way we think, feel, and express emotions is linked to the pain's development. And learning to reframe our thinking can greatly impact how we experience pain, as well.

For this reason, somatic exercises are often used in integrative health centers to help manage and treat chronic pain. Somatic therapies are about listening to the body as well as the mind. This follows in the footsteps of ancient traditions like traditional Chinese medicine, which use the mind–body connection to understand our vitality and health.

Mind-Body Connection

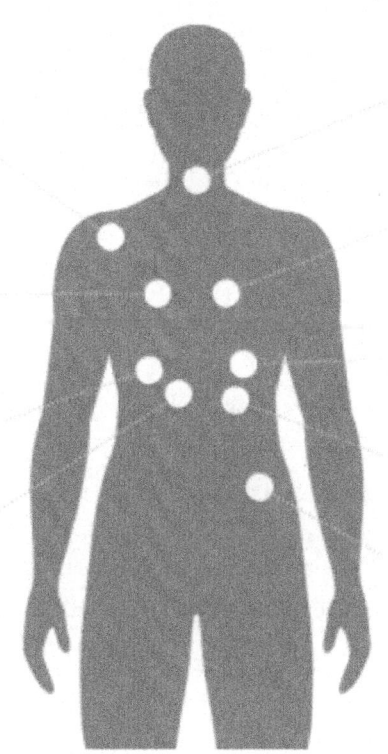

BACK & SHOULDERS - BURDEN
Feeling the pressure of responsibility, overwhelm and stress. Manifests as physical tension.

LUNGS - GRIEF/SADNESS
Suppressed feelings of grief can lead to respiratory issues and a weakened immune system.

LIVER - ANGER/RAGE
Irritability, frustration, and anger. Chronic anger can weaken liver function.

KIDNEYS - FEAR
Chronic fear or anxiety can lead to fatigue and low back pain.

THROAT - EXPRESSING VOICE
Challenges speaking personal truth or communicating feelings or emotions.

HEART - JOY
When balanced, promotes joy and emotional stability. Imbalance leads to excessive excitement, insomnia, anxiety.

SPLEEN - OVERTHINKING
Excessive mental activity such as worry can lead to digestive issues and fatigue.

STOMACH - WORRY/ANXIETY
Chronic anxiety can lead to digestive problems.

HIPS & PSOAS - FEAR/STRESS
Unresolved fear and anxiety can lead to chronic tension in hips and psoas.

As a trauma-informed somatic practitioner and mindful movement teacher, I am passionate about making resources like this more accessible. After all, not everyone has access to individual therapy, whether due to financial or healthcare insecurity. These boundaries keep many from getting the help they need. Books like this can fill some of that gap.

Even if you have access to therapy, it's often just one hour a week at best. That still leaves a lot of hours in the week when you need support. The exercises that I introduce in this book are a self-therapy you can practice when you're on your own.

To put it simply, I wrote this book with the aim of helping you help *you*.

Experience is the best teacher. And the exercises in this book are an essential part of understanding somatic therapy. This book presents various exercises, some of which are best suited for beginners, while others are more intermediate. Treat them like experiments and as opportunities to learn more about yourself. Some exercises will resonate with you; others won't. And that's *okay*. We all approach things differently.

I want to note that these practices might not be for everyone. It is possible that they'll bring up difficult emotions, so it's crucial to be gentle with yourself. Ease into these practices. Start by dipping your toe in. Move at your own pace, and don't feel pressured to rush the process. This isn't a race, and there is no distinct "finish line."

I also want to manage your expectations. This is meant to be a journey, not a quick fix. These exercises are stepping stones on your healing journey, but you might not notice progress at first. It takes consistency and practice. Start small when incorporating these practices into your life, and build up. Here are some tips to help you start this journey:

1. If you're anything like me, you might be tempted to skip ahead to the juiciest parts of the book. But I encourage you to read the book in order.

2. Once you've done a few exercises from "Body Awareness" and "Grounding," feel free to then work through the book nonsequentially.

3. The workbook exercises are there to help you process and better understand the principles laid out in the exercises. I highly encourage you to do those exercises. If you don't want to write in the book, feel free to write in a notebook or journal.

4. Once you find the exercises that resonate with you, continue to practice them. As you do, you will find that your experience will deepen. New insights and understanding might arise. Tune into them.

It is my goal to bring your mind–body connection to a place of harmony. For many, stress, illness, or trauma has taught them that it is not safe to truly connect with and inhabit their body. These exercises will help you rediscover a sense of safety and peace within your body.

Go at your own pace, be gentle with yourself, and stick to what resonates. I can't promise you that at the end of this book you'll be healed. But I can assure you that learning these tools will help you on your way.

Part 1:
The Foundational Pillars

The Principles of Somatic Therapy

The human body is not an instrument to be used, but a realm of one's being to be experienced, explored, enriched and, thereby, educated. –Thomas Hanna, founder of Clinical Somatic Education

To truly understand something, you should start with the very foundation of it. Somatic therapy is no different. Before you get into practicing some of the exercises, it would benefit you to have a firm grasp of what somatic therapy is all about. Knowing the core meaning and purpose of somatic therapy will allow you to pursue the exercises more intentionally.

Definition of Somatic Therapy

Let's start with the basic definition of somatic therapy. Though we discussed it briefly in the Introduction, taking a deeper dive will provide a better understanding. Simply put, somatic therapy is a type of holistic approach to healing that brings focus to the connection between mind and body. At its core, it builds from the principle that our bodies hold onto emotions, memories, and trauma, affecting our mental and physical well-being.

Through exercises like physical awareness and listening deeply, we can process any tension, trauma, or difficult emotions while also gaining insight into our experiences. This helps us disentangle our stories and gain valuable insights into our emotional responses.

These insights can then be used to approach how we think and feel about our experiences. Somatic therapy emphasizes healing as a holistic and integrative process that involves both the mind *and* the body. Powerful stuff, with incredible applications.

The Evolution of Somatics

To understand the somatic modality better, we should take a brief look at the roots of the practice. At its core, somatic therapy is similar to holistic approaches taught by various ancient cultures, and it often incorporates them. From the Indigenous peoples of North America to ancient China, there is a rich history of cultures understanding the mind–body connection long before modern somatic therapy was developed.

However, modern somatic therapy is commonly traced back to various therapeutic practices from the early 20th century, heavily influenced by pioneers like Wilhelm Reich, who explored the connection between our body and our emotions in greater depth. It was in the 1960s and

1970s that figures like Alexander Lowen developed bioenergetics, which focused on bodywork and breathing techniques.

Eventually, the term "somatic" came about through the integration of psychology and body awareness. It then gained popularity throughout the 1980s and 1990s. During this time, researchers and therapists alike were studying the importance of the body in emotional healing. Today, modern somatic therapy includes a range of techniques that are ever-evolving. As our understanding of psychology and physiology develops, so does somatic therapy.

Some of the incredible body-centered techniques that influence somatic therapy, and are often incorporated into it, are:

- somatic experiencing
- Hakomi method
- Alexander technique
- Rolfing structural integration
- qigong and tai chi
- Feldenkrais method

This history shows a major shift from purely cognitive therapies to those that incorporate the body. These techniques are more effective in healing, as they are less about overanalyzing and overthinking. Instead, they allow us to simply feel and process what our mind and body are trying to tell us.

The Role of Trauma

As I mentioned in the Introduction, trauma is not an event. It's not something that occurs. It is something that dwells within us following a traumatic event. It is how we think, feel, and act as a result of an event that has shaken us to our core. Understanding this gives us greater power over the impact.

What many don't realize is that trauma is also stored physically in the body. The lasting imprint of trauma can rewrite how your brain and nervous system function, causing tension and physical symptoms like body aches and headaches. Sometimes, physical ailments occur within the body, such as obesity, heart attack, diabetes, and even cancer (Harvard Health Publishing, 2023).

The human nervous system is the basis of communication for the human body. It carries electrical signals between our body and our mind using a complex system of neurons that span our entire body and brain. It takes our internal thoughts and makes them into actions; it takes external stimuli and creates experiences and memories. For this reason, it plays a crucial role in somatic practice. This modality strives to regulate and calm the nervous system, allowing relief from trauma impact.

For many of us with trauma, the fear and discomfort can come down to a feeling of not feeling safe within our own body. After all, experience has taught us that. Whether the trauma is physical or emotional, it can present and reinforce this idea over time, leaving us wanting to disconnect. We associate any inner experience with unsafety, which is a huge problem—because there's nowhere to go! We can't escape our body and ourselves. Somatic therapy presents and reinforces the idea that we can feel safe within our bodies by making room for little pockets of safety every day. Regulating your nervous system requires safety, so ensure that you are listening to your body and taking things at your own pace.

Body Awareness

Somatic therapy modalities increase our awareness and safety within our own bodies. In reconnecting with our physical senses and experiences, we calm our nervous system, allowing for healing to begin. So, how does this work?

First of all, let's talk about the disconnect that many of us have with our bodies. As previously mentioned, there's a safety concern. Traumatic events and our responses to them have made us believe that our own body is a danger zone. But there's nothing we can do to escape our body and, at best, we wind up dysregulated.

Somatic therapy calls attention to bodily sensations. It encourages us to heighten our awareness of them. This, in turn, fosters emotional processing and healing. Be prepared to feel some pretty big emotions when you start working with somatic healing exercises. When we begin to listen to our bodies, we start to hear and understand the emotions and trauma stored within us.

Our bodies are a source of wisdom. That might sound like a platitude, but it's true. Everything our body does is designed to protect us and keep us safe. When we are able to listen to what our bodies are telling us, we start to understand and move toward healing and harmony. Moreover, it cultivates a better understanding of the physical sensations we feel. Ancient traditions such as Taoism and Buddhism have taught us that physical sensations correlate with emotional states. So, when we learn to listen to our bodies, we are also understanding our emotional existence.

Benefits of Somatic Therapy

Emotional Release

Through somatic exercises, you will learn to express and process emotions that were previously trapped in your body. Imagine all the stress, tension, and grief leaving your body. It can be incredibly cathartic and fosters a much healthier emotional landscape by allowing for vulnerability and expression.

What you might be avoiding the most—feeling your feelings—is what can and *will* help you heal. Opening yourself up to feeling what you need to feel can help you process and release emotions. This lightens your load and enhances how you function overall. This isn't about improving one piece of the puzzle. It's about a widespread change throughout your entire nervous system.

Carrying around these "trapped" emotions in our bodies can be an intense strain on our nervous system. Allowing for emotional release through somatic exercises allows for the nervous system to gain balance. Our body needs to "even the scales" when it's holding onto all that emotional energy, and that often means increasing inflammation and muscle tension in the body to compensate (Murnan, 2023). Releasing the emotions also means allowing for some of those more negative impacts to fall by the wayside.

Here's an inventory of emotions that you can refer to throughout this book:

Wheel of Emotions

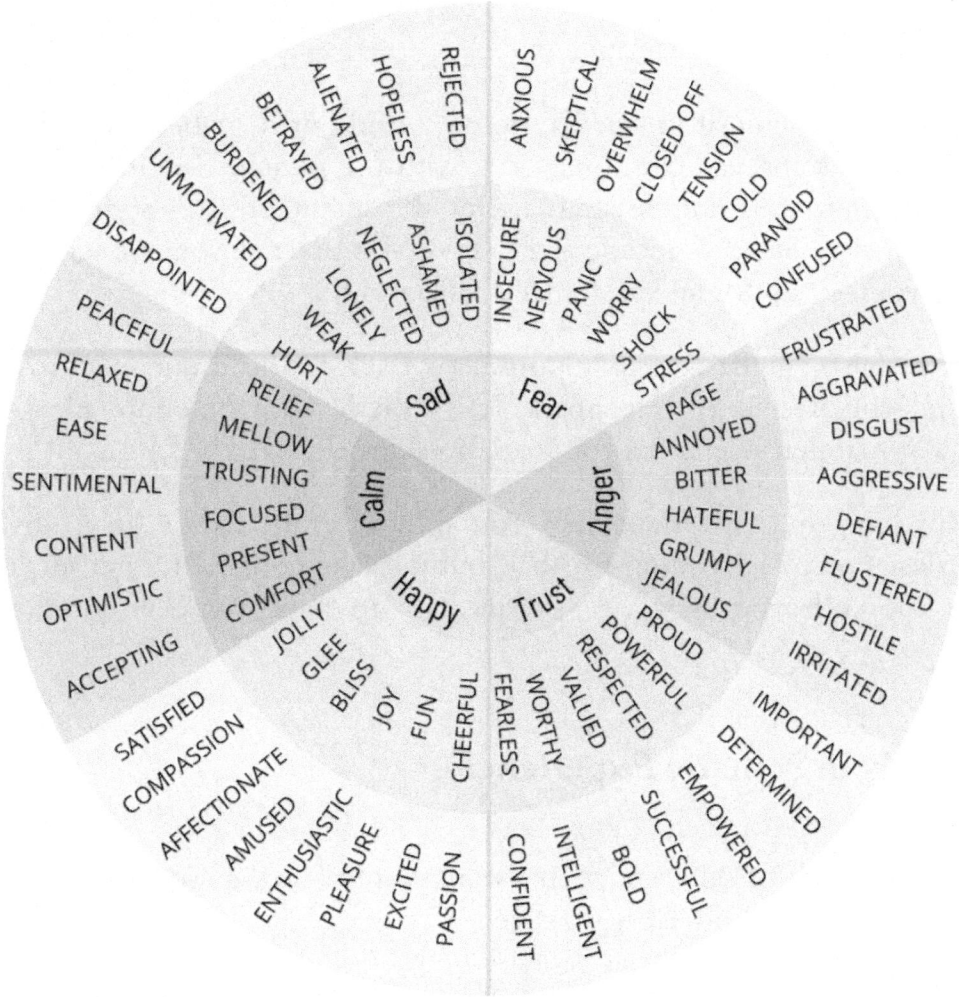

Nervous System Regulation

Many of these techniques directly promote relaxation and stress relief. Somatic practices help activate the parasympathetic nervous system. The parasympathetic nervous system, if you are unfamiliar with it, regulates involuntary bodily functions when our bodies are at rest. It generally promotes relaxation, digestion, and energy conservation. This is accomplished by slowing our heart rate, increasing intestinal activity, and stimulating glandular secretions. The parasympathetic nervous system counteracts the effects of the sympathetic nervous system, responsible for the "fight-or-flight" response.

The parasympathetic nervous system, in other words, gives us a chance to rest and "chill out." But I don't want you to think that there will never be moments of discomfort. Bringing harmony to your nervous systems doesn't mean you'll never again be dysregulated or uncomfortable. However, it will give you a feeling of empowerment to respond appropriately to that discomfort.

Best Quality of Life

Emotional resilience is crucial in our day-to-day. Without it, it becomes all too easy to be discouraged by life's setbacks. You don't "roll with the punches" quite as well, and that can leave you feeling burdened and frustrated. But the integration of body and mind leads to sustained emotional resilience—meaning the more you practice somatic techniques, the more you are setting yourself up for an emotionally resilient life.

Somatic exercises also emphasize the importance of self-care and ongoing growth. Self-care is not some indulgent lifestyle of selfishness. It is exactly what it sounds like—taking care of yourself. Regular maintenance keeps you from breaking down over time.

More than anything, it is my hope that you find a return to joy and satisfaction. These exercises are designed to set you up for that, but it'll take consistency and dedication. As you venture into this endeavor, however, I want you to have some important tools at your disposal.

Three Methods in Somatic Experiencing

There are three methods of self-regulation I want you to know as you embark on this journey. You can apply them to any and every practice:

- **Titration:** It's important that you approach trauma in manageable amounts. After all, we don't want you getting overwhelmed. Titration allows you to confront trauma without that happening. It calls for taking things slow and steady. Don't feel the need to jump into the deep end too soon. And don't feel you have to do it too frequently, either—that can be counterproductive. Instead, break your trauma down into digestible pieces and go from there.

- **Pendulation:** This process consists of alternating between discomfort and comfort. When we practice pendulation, we are reinforcing the body's ability to self-regulate and shift between states, enhancing resilience. As it fosters a sense of safety, it allows you to explore discomfort in a more controlled manner. It also empowers you to regain control over your healing journey.

- **Resourcing:** Resourcing is looking for the rainbows, so to speak. This technique involves identifying and recalling specific resources—supportive people, safe places, calming activities—that will provide safety and comfort during times of distress. When we incorporate these resources into therapeutic sessions, we enhance our sense of safety, helping us learn to better self-regulate.

I want to briefly mention an important concept in somatic therapy and trauma therapy, and that is productive pain vs. harmful pain. In other words, learn to recognize which sensations are productive (giving us information) and which ones are harmful. Any sudden sharp pain, for instance, is typically harmful and unnecessary. Be sure to step away from an activity if it is bringing up unhelpful sensations.

Throughout the course of this book, you can refer to this inventory of sensations. Ask yourself—what's the felt sense experience I'm having?

Body Sensations Inventory

CALM	BURNING	QUIVERING	RACING
SETTLED	SHAKING	PULLING	PLEASURE
STILL	SHIVERING	KNOTS	SLEEPY
STRONG	RESTLESS	WIRY	PULSING
FLOWING	TREMBLING	NUMBING	PRESSURE
EASE	VIBRATING	HEAVY	PRICKLY
OPEN	HOT	BUBBLY	CONTRACTING
LIGHT	CHILLS	ELECTRIC	TIGHT
TENDER	COLD	AGITATED	TENSE
ALIVE	TWISTING	SPINNING	PINS & NEEDLES
VIBRANT	PAIN	SORE	BRUISING
FLUTTERING	CHURNING	EXPANDING	HOLLOW

Things You Should Know

Before we begin the exercises, here are some important steps to follow for every exercise:

1. **Go inward:** No matter the exercise, bring your awareness and attention inward. If you need to, close your eyes to encourage this.

2. **Move slowly:** You don't need to move fast in any of the exercises. In slowing down, you are getting a better sense of what's happening in your body.

3. **Allow:** Recognize any strong sensations in your body that call for attention. You don't need to change the sensations. Just allow them to be. Breathe gently. From this place of mindfulness, you can make adjustments to make yourself more comfortable, rather than having a knee-jerk reaction to get comfortable. Notice the difference.

4. **Identify:** What are your feelings? Refer back to the diagrams of sensations and emotions. Invite a curiosity to these feelings.

5. **Choose a response:** From this place of pause, spaciousness, and curiosity, begin to perform the exercise. Do so in the way that suits you best. And in life, respond to what's happening somatically. Make sure you do so in a way that serves you and doesn't harm you.

As Viktor Frankl (n.d.) said, "Between stimulus and response, there is a space. In that space lies our freedom and our power to choose our response. In our response lies our growth and our happiness."

You are taking an incredible first step in your healing journey. These exercises will be wonderful tools for you to process and release the trauma that dwells within your mind and body. As you turn the page and head into the next part, remember: Take what serves you. Leave the rest. You've got this.

Part 2:
Somatic Exercises

Body Awareness

In this section, we start to dive into the exercises. As mentioned previously, it is highly recommended that you start here. These exercises give you a firm foundation to build success in somatic techniques. Once you get past the section on grounding, feel free to skip around, keeping in mind that some techniques are best suited for intermediate practitioners.

As you go through each exercise, make sure that you are slowing down to spend time with your body. That's what somatic exercises are really all about. They nudge you toward awareness of certain areas in your body. Throughout these techniques, you will become more aware of sensations and changes in your body so that you are able to shift and release them.

Talk therapy only goes so far and, with certain topics, might not be as effective as we hoped. Somatics is different in that it requires you to *feel* your way toward healing. It often makes the journey a lot more manageable and empowering, and less analytical.

Exercise 1: Body Scan

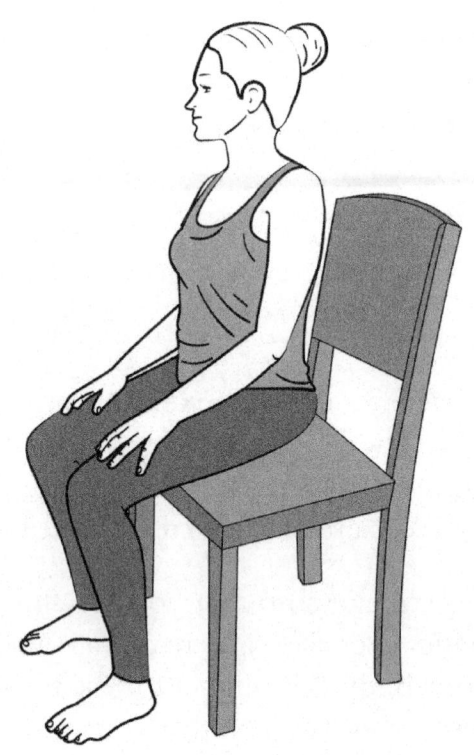

Level: Beginner

Imagine a laser copier scanning and understanding each part of your body. That's a bit what a body scan is like. Through mindfulness, meditation, and body awareness, you scan yourself from the crown of your head to your feet. This exercise allows you to be more cognizant of the feelings and sensations that you are experiencing. It also gives you the opportunity to release any held tension or stress.

Not only can this be a peaceful and mindful experience, but recent studies have found that even taking a few moments to do a quick body scan can significantly lower the severity and perception of chronic pain (Cleveland Clinic, 2023). It's also a great way to train your nervous system to relax. The more you practice this technique, the more predisposed your nervous system is to relax (Cleveland Clinic, 2023). Let's get into it!

1. **Find a comfortable position:** This particular exercise can be done in pretty much any position as long as you are comfortable, be that lying down, sitting, or standing up.

2. **Close your eyes:** If you don't feel comfortable closing your eyes, you can also try lowering your gaze or focusing on a single spot.

3. **Take a few deep, even breaths:** Take these breaths in through the nose and out through the mouth. Focus on the sensation of each breath, and relax into your body.

4. **Begin at the top of your body:** Focus in on the sensations you feel in your head. Is there any pain or tension? Pulsing? Don't try to judge or change any of the feelings. Simply acknowledge them.

5. **Move down your body:** Whenever you're comfortable, begin to slowly move down your body, taking time to focus on each part—your neck and shoulders, your torso and arms, and then your legs. What sensations do you feel? Notice and acknowledge them before moving to the next body part.

6. **Finish at your feet:** Finish off the body scan at your feet, going all the way to your toes.

7. **Finish off the scan softly and gradually:** Return your attention to your surroundings while taking a slow, deep breath. Note how you feel.

Workbook Exercises

1. How did it feel to tune into your body, one piece at a time? What sensations did you notice?

2. How did you feel after the exercise, as opposed to before it?

Exercise 2: Understanding Misuse vs. Proper Use

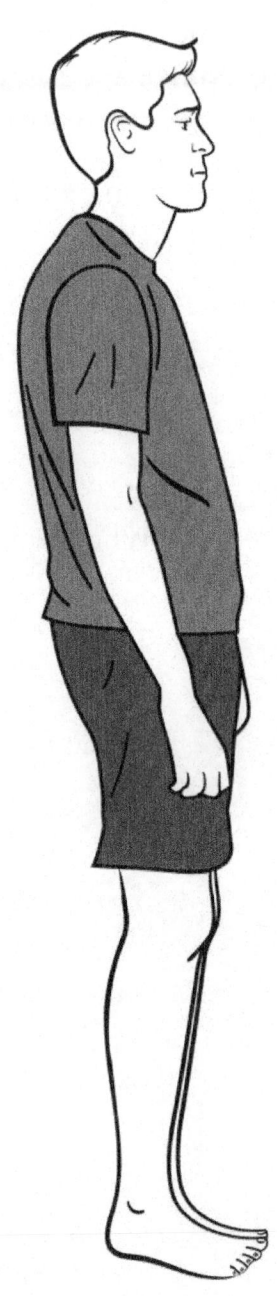
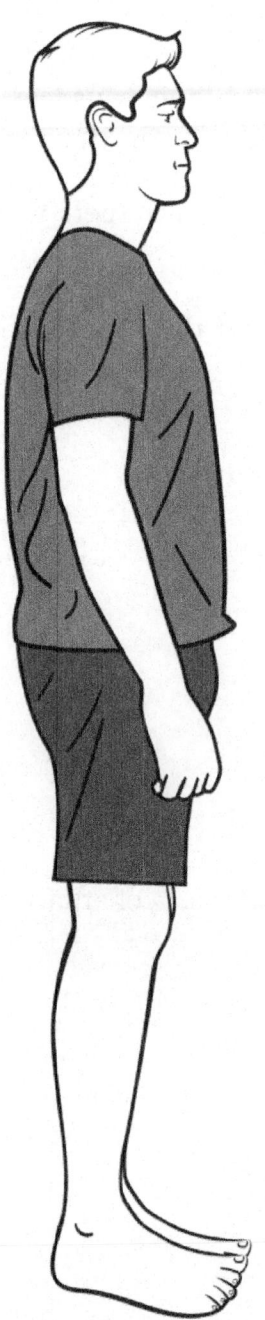

Level: Beginner

To the outsider, this might seem like a simple standing exercise. But for the person practicing it, this is a powerful body exercise. Understanding the difference between misuse and proper use is incredibly important when we are reconnecting with our bodies through somatic exercises.

Believe it or not, our posture has a significant impact on our neurological and cognitive function. This is, in large part, due to the salient network. This network responds to various inputs, such as biofeedback and physiological mechanisms, and, in turn, influences everything from emotions to intellectual performance (*How Posture Affects Neurological and Cognitive Function*, 2024). By correcting your posture, you are actually helping your brain!

1. **Begin the exercise by standing:** Before you get into the fine details of the exercise, take a moment to just stand. Notice and acknowledge the downward pull of gravity. Is it an overall pull, or do you feel it more strongly in certain areas?

2. **Stand in front of a mirror:** Now, for this exercise you want to be able to see yourself. Move to a mirror and notice your standing stance.

3. **Try doing common components of misuse:** To really understand misuse in the body, try doing the following, observing how they feel and how they look in the mirror:

    a. your head tilted back

    b. your neck and chin both tilted forward

    c. your upper chest falling back or caving in

    d. an arched lower back with your pelvis thrust forward

    e. knees locked

    f. leaning forward on the balls of your feet or toes

    g. shoulders going up with each inhale and down with each exhale

4. **Notice and ask questions:** As you are deliberately standing in misuse, ask yourself, "How do I feel after demonstrating misuse? Do these movements feel familiar? Were any of these recognizable as habits?"

5. **Take a deep breath and a short walk:** To clear your mind and body, take a few deep breaths and take a short, brisk walk around the room.

6. **Return to the mirror and explore proper use:** Now that you've explored misuse, it's time to demonstrate proper use in front of the mirror:

a. your head a touch upward and forward, poised right above the spine

   b. neck slightly back but not completely straightened out

   c. lengthen and widen your back, from your hip sockets to the top of the spine

   d. unlock your legs and place your weight on your heels

   e. arms loose at your sides

   f. ribs should move in and out with your breath

7. **Notice and ask questions:** Notice how you feel in your body and ask, "How do I feel? Was that awkward? Natural? How is my shape in the mirror? Do I look and/or feel different?"

Workbook Exercises

1. How did it feel to intentionally put your body into misuse? Did you notice at any time that your habits are similar to the misuse?

2. How did you feel after adjusting your body with proper use? Did it feel natural? Awkward? Notice if any pain in your body was reduced.

Exercise 3: Lessening Effort

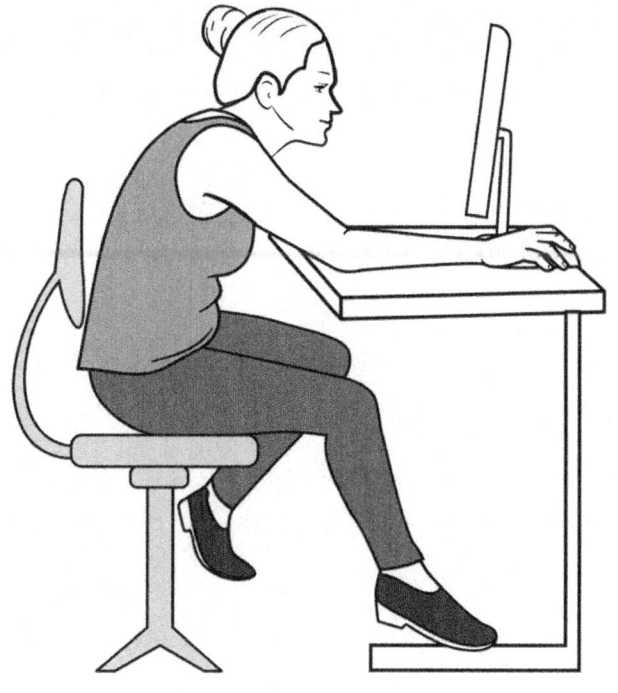

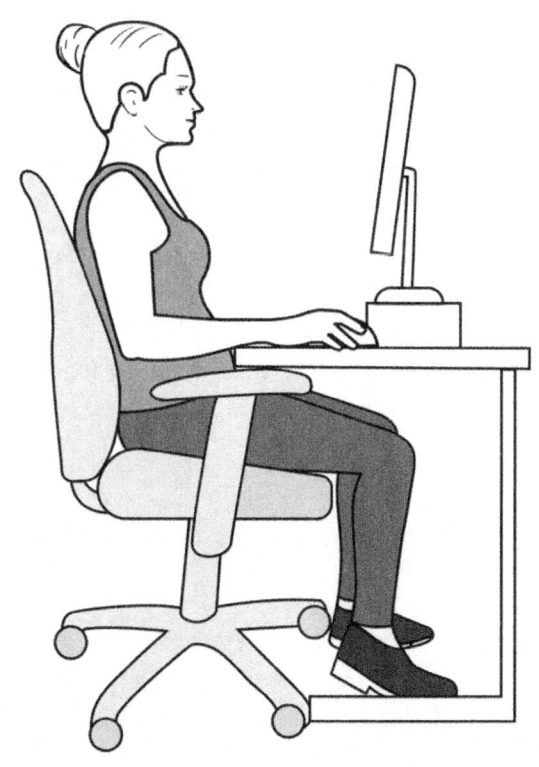

Level: Beginner

In somatic therapy, excessive or unnecessary tension is often a sign that there is an imbalance in the body that is affecting the mind. The more you can become aware of this tension and address it, the more effective your practice will be on this journey of somatic healing.

Ask yourself, "How can I do this with less effort?" More often than not, less is more.

1. **Sit at a desk in front of a computer or laptop:** As you type, notice how you hold yourself and how you type.

2. **Ask yourself a question:** Pay attention. Are you tapping the keys hard? If so, try asking yourself if you can do less. Could you get away with tapping the keys more lightly?

3. **Tap the keys with less force:** If so, tap the keys with less force. Keep asking yourself if you can do less, until the answer is no.

4. **Pay attention to how you are sitting:** Is there tension in your muscles? Are you hunched over? Straighten your spine and loosen the muscles, holding yourself as lightly as possible.

5. **Continue to do so until you are using the least amount of effort possible:** Again, keep asking yourself if you can do less. Do this until the answer is, eventually, no.

Workbook Exercises

1. What did you notice when lessening the effort? What sensations did you feel?

2. How could you apply this activity to whatever activity you do (e.g., running, walking, sitting, etc.)?

Exercise 4: Lying-Down Work

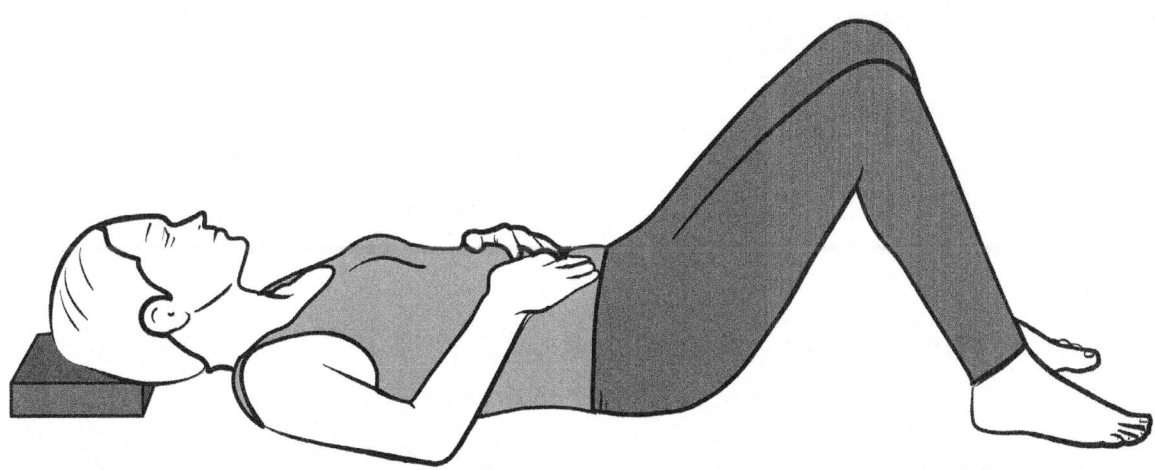

Level: Beginner

This somatic exercise is pretty common among actors. This is, in part, due to its conception by a Shakespearian actor, who accidentally made a discovery while trying to figure out why he kept losing his voice after performances. He discovered that there was a link between his posture, how tense his muscles were before speech, and how often he lost his voice.

Lying-down work is based on the Alexander technique and its efficacy is backed by science. A recent study was done that discovered regular use of the Alexander technique lessened the rate of neck pain in subjects over a 12-month period (Selhub, 2015). Let's get into lying-down work ourselves!

1. **Lie down on the floor:** With your back on the (carpeted) floor or a mat, and your head elevated by a one- to two-inch-thick book, bend your knees gently. Don't pull them together. Your feet should still be flat on the floor, set somewhat apart. Rest your hands on your abdomen and allow the floor to hold you.

2. **Bring your attention inward:** Start to notice what is going on inside of you. Is there any excess tension? Are you holding your breath? Is your mind racing about everything you need to do today? *Notice* what is going on inside yourself, but don't attempt to change anything.

3. **Say these statements aloud:** As you allow the ground to support you, begin saying these statements aloud:

    a. "Let my neck be free."

    b. "Let my head release away from my spine and body."

    c. "Let my back lengthen and widen, setting free my bones, muscles, and nervous system."

    d. "Let my knees aim toward the ceiling, allowing for more space in the joints of my hips and ankles."

    e. "As I let my ankles release, let my heels drop to the floor and my feet spread out on the floor."

4. **Repeat statements A–C.**

5. **Say these statements aloud:** "Let my shoulders release from my back. My elbows will now release from my shoulders, and my wrists from my elbows."

6. **Repeat statements A–C again.**

7. **Say these statements aloud:** "Let my hips lift gently and lower back down to the floor. As my hips lower, let my back lengthen."

8. **Repeat statements A–C.**

Workbook Exercises

1. Do you feel your back more?

2. If yes, what do you notice in your back when this happens?

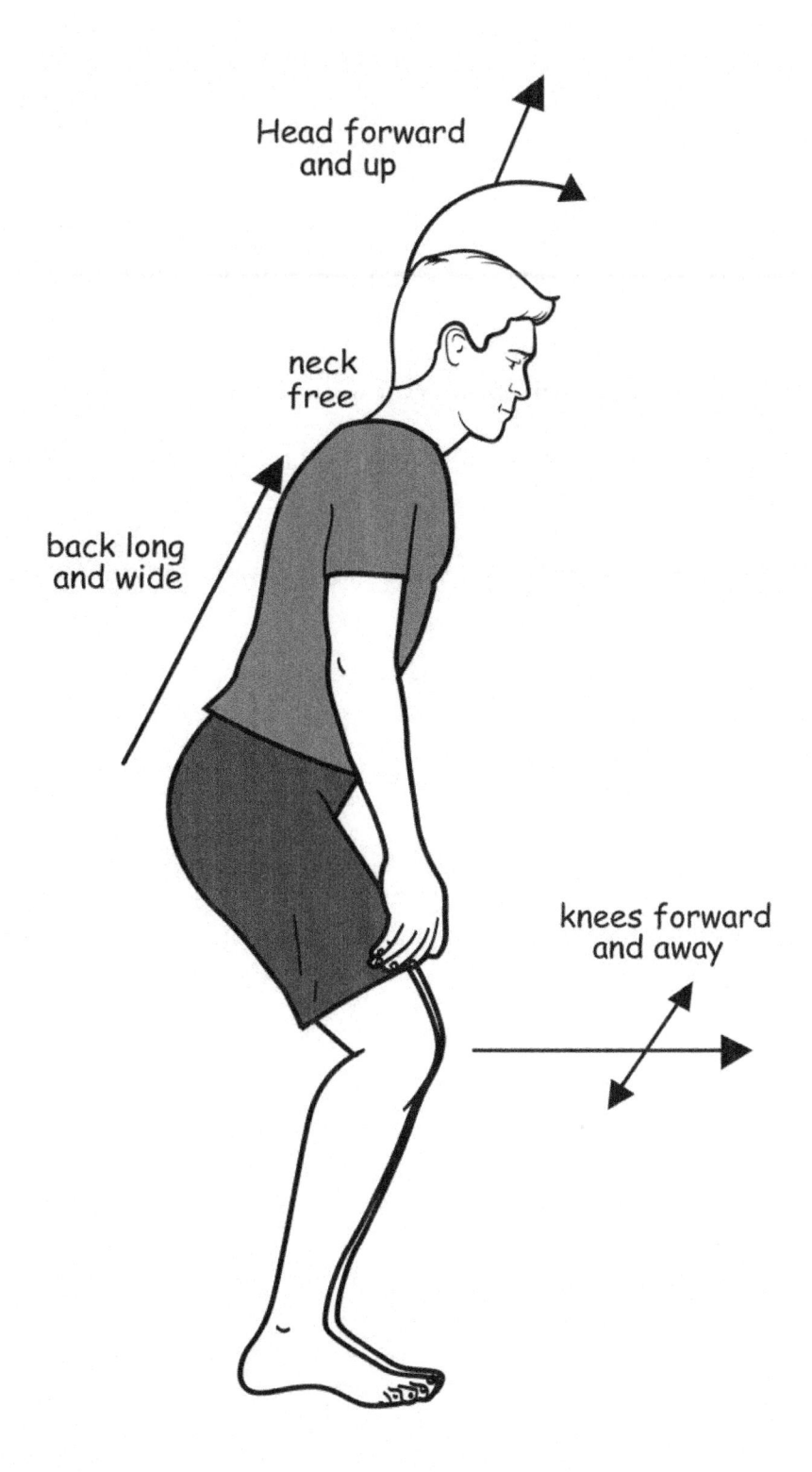

Exercise 5: Monkey Stance

Level: Beginner

The Monkey Stance is a unique exercise, as it is an incredibly common stance seen in small children but also a foundational exercise of the Alexander technique. Something that comes so naturally to young kids is something that takes a little extra effort on our part. This exercise stylizes the posture and movement to help you regain, or even find, the hinging movement of your hip joints, as well as allowing your spine to maintain its full length when leaning forward. This simple but powerful exercise grounds you within your body as well as to the ground, while still allowing for free movement.

1. **Begin this exercise standing.**

2. **Now, allow your knees to release and move slightly forward:** As they bend, let them move slightly apart from each other.

3. **Release your hips, ankles, and hips:** You want them loose and free.

4. **With your head directed forward and up, pivot your hips forward:** As you do this, ensure your heels are bearing your weight.

5. **Allow your arms hang loosely by your sides:** As you breathe, allow your shoulders to widen.

6. **Slowly lower yourself in place:** Do this by bending your knees and pivoting forward. This is the simple Monkey Stance.

7. **Continue bending your knees and pivoting forward:** This would then be the deeper Monkey Stance.

8. **Try moving from this stance into other activities:** You should feel the support of the ground coming up through your legs and torso, and connecting all the way through your arms.

Workbook Exercises

1. How did you feel before doing the Monkey Stance exercise?

2. How did your body feel during the Monkey Stance exercise?

_____

_____

_____

3. How did your body feel afterward?

Exercise 6: Supportive Touch

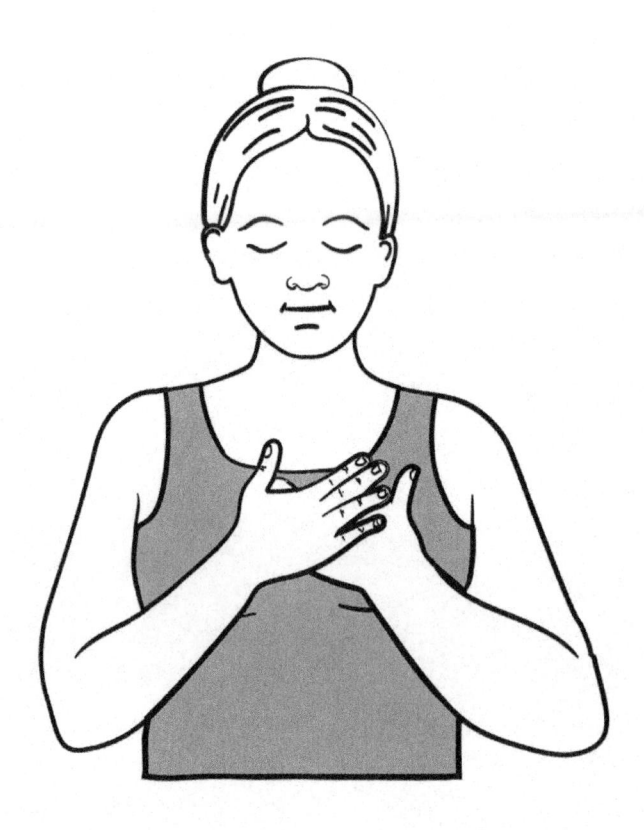

Level: Beginner

This is a great point to recognize and acknowledge that self-compassion is the key to all of the exercises in this book. I'd go so far as to say that it is absolutely crucial to the somatic modality itself. You can't hate yourself into change—at least, not effective and meaningful change. Showing yourself kindness on your journey is the best path forward.

This exercise, created by Dr. Kristen Neff, is designed to create an awareness of what feels safe and nourishing. It can be done lying down, sitting, or even standing. Remember to invite love and compassion into yourself, especially if deep or heavy emotions come up. If those feelings do come up, remember to stop, allow, and get curious. However, if the emotions prove to be too intense, refer back to the titration and pendulation strategies mentioned earlier in this book.

One of the best ways to stop and care for yourself in moments when emotions rise up is through supportive touch. This simple exercise has a profound impact on the nervous system and your state of mind. By activating the care and parasympathetic nervous systems, touch—be it from others or yourself—supports you to calm down. It also helps you feel safe in the moment. Next time you feel overwhelmed, try this exercise and see how you feel afterward.

1. Should you notice you're under stress, take two to three deep, refreshing breaths.

2. Gently rest your hand over your heart. Take notice of the gentle pressure and warmth of your hand. Depending on how you feel, you might want to consider placing both hands over your heart.

3. If you wish, try making small circles over your heart with each breath in and each breath out.

4. Stay with that feeling as long for as feels comfortable—for as long as you like.

5. If you feel uneasy about placing your hand over your heart, experiment with other locations on the body, such as:

   - a hand placed on your cheek
   - stroking your arms gently
   - a hand on your abdomen
   - cupping one hand in the other while both are in your lap

6. Continue to practice this exercise regularly. As you do so, it will become second nature to comfort yourself as needed.

Workbook Exercises

1. How did you feel after participating in this activity?

2. Was there any discomfort? How can you respond to that?

Grounding

Now that we have focused some time and energy on body awareness, I want to move on to another important exercise type—grounding. Simply put, grounding is the ability to find and maintain connection with the earth and one's own body. This type of exercise is incredibly important when dealing with stress and trauma. When we become dysregulated by diving into those areas, grounding can be a bit like hitting the reboot button. It draws us back into what is real. It also gives us the ability to tune into our body's messaging and needs.

Grounding isn't just a way to stay connected, however. It also activates the parasympathetic nervous system, flooding our system with relaxation and peace. It has been shown scientifically that standing with our feet on the earth (a classic grounding technique) begins to relax our muscles, causing a noticeable shift in parasympathetic functioning—slower breathing, slower heart rate, and so on (HYNS Team, 2023). Practicing this alongside body awareness will help you get more out of each exercise.

Exercise 7: Squeeze Hug

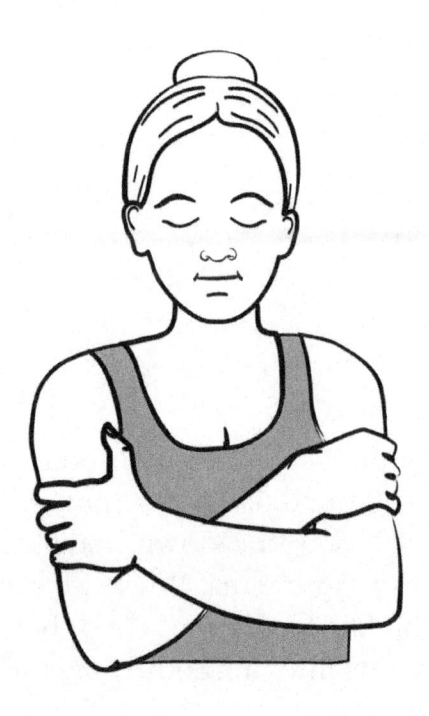

Level: Beginner

This exercise is simple in execution but can have an incredible impact on the nervous system. The Squeeze Hug is a great way to self-regulate when you are feeling anxious. It can also help you break out of the freeze response that you may have developed as a result of trauma. Often, when we experience these things, we disconnect and dissociate from our bodies. But this exercise can reconnect us to our bodies and the natural healing mechanisms that it possesses.

1. **Cross your arms across your chest:** As you do so, place each hand on the opposite arm.

2. **Squeeze:** Squeeze your body with your arms, pulling your arms around yourself as hard as is comfortable for you. It's like you're giving yourself a tight hug.

3. **Maintain as long as necessary:** Continue to squeeze, giving yourself this hug until you feel more regulated.

4. **(Optional) Breathe in and out deeply:** Take deep breaths as you do this activity, adding to its relaxing properties.

5. **(Optional) Flex and unflex your back:** While not necessary, this can also add some relaxation and extra movement to your spine, furthering the relaxation.

6. **With your breath, pull your arms in and gently squeeze each arm with the opposite hand as you do so:** This allows for a gentle tense-and-relax motion that can regulate the nervous system and reconnect you with your body.

7. **Notice how your body feels:** Check in with your body and the present moment. Remind yourself that, here and now, you are safe.

Workbook Exercises

1. How did you feel before the exercise? What was on your mind?

2. As you checked in at the end of the exercise, what did you notice? Did you feel safer? Why or why not?

Exercise 8: Tuning Into the Senses

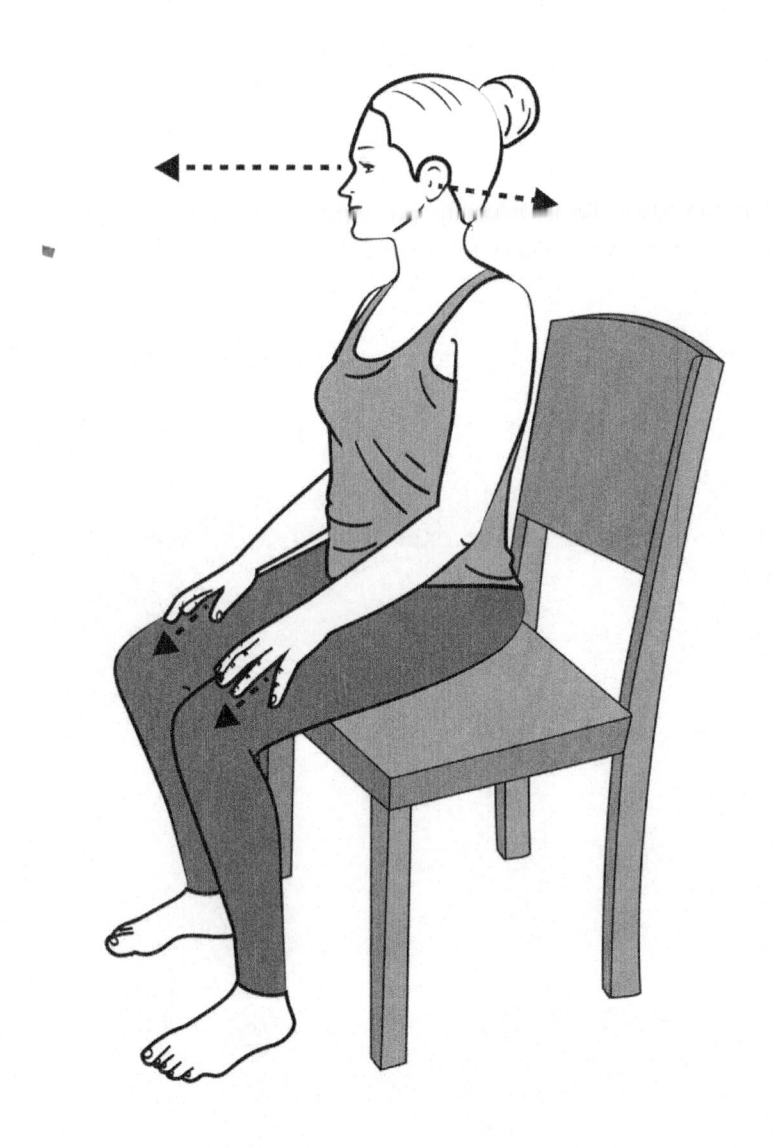

Level: Beginner

This exercise trains your body to trigger the parasympathetic response by using a grounding technique. Throughout this book, we've discussed the importance of our nervous system in regulating our emotions and responses. The sympathetic and parasympathetic nervous systems both play their part, but when things are out of balance, we sometimes need to correct them through gentle grounding and awareness. When the sympathetic nervous system activates, you are more alert and aware. But you are also often more tense. While this can be good when you are running from a lion, it's unnecessary when you're sitting in traffic. The parasympathetic nervous system has a more calming role.

To be healthy in today's world, we want to have a more parasympathetic-dominant nervous system. A great way to accomplish this is by intentionally grounding our body in our senses. This exercise helps us do that. For you to relax, you need to receive a message from your body that you *are* safe. Connecting to the present moment and your body through your senses is a great way to accomplish this.

1. **To begin, take a comfortable, calming breath:** When you are ready, it's time to open your awareness to the moment and space around you.

2. **Touch—touch three things in your environment:** As you do this, describe each item in your mind. For example, you might touch the table in front of you and think, *This is cold and hard.*

3. **Sight—look around and notice three things that you can see:** Describe those three items in your mind as well.

4. **Hearing—notice three different sources of sound:** Maybe it's the air-conditioning running, or the sounds of cars outside. In your mind, describe what they sound like.

5. **Notice how your body feels:** Check in with your body as you become more centered in this moment.

Workbook Exercises

1. What did you notice about your body's response to tuning into your senses?

2. Which sense was hardest for you to connect to? Why do you think that is?

Exercise 9: Standing in Your Power

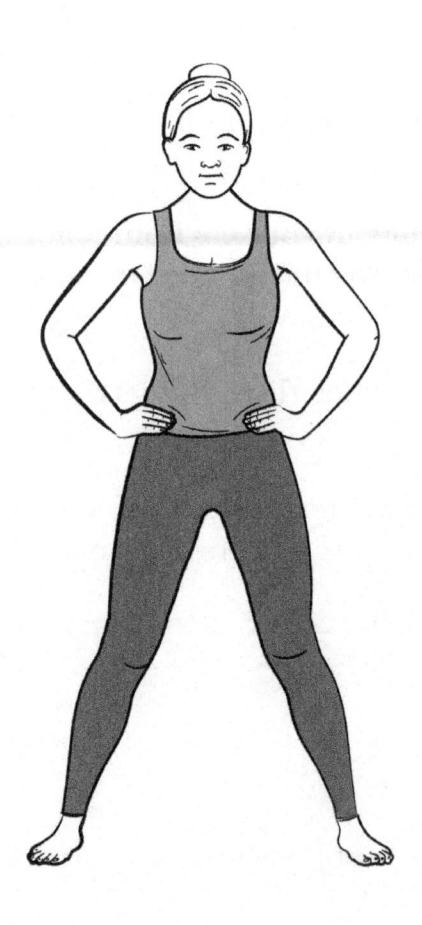

Level: Beginner

Posture has a profound impact on our cognitive and emotional functioning. Think about it for a moment. When you are feeling stressed or insecure, you might shrink in on yourself—shoulders hunched, eyes downcast. Eventually, it has a bit of a Pavlovian effect. When you adopt that stance, it's like a switch flips in your brain, letting you know it's time to be insecure and anxious. By adopting a more powerful stance, we can train our brains to think and feel more powerful and self-assured (Loncar, 2021).

Power poses stem from research that began back in 2010 and sought to uncover whether brief postural adjustments would make a psychological, behavioral, or hormonal impact. What the researchers found were nonverbal factors that played a part in us feeling powerful (or, conversely, powerless) (Loncar, 2021). By adjusting our posture to reflect a positive attitude, we encourage that positive attitude to occur.

1. **Start by collapsing your back:** Hunch over and make yourself as small as possible. You want to embody a limp rag—like you can't even hold yourself up.

2. **Notice how that stance affects your breathing:** Pause and notice.

3. **Notice how it impacts your feelings and mood.**

4. **Be aware of your body:** Pause and consider for a moment what it feels like to be small, hunched over, and collapsed in on yourself.

5. **Say, "I am powerful":** Do this while still hunched over.

6. **Say, "I am happy":** Remain hunched over while saying this.

7. **Notice if you feel those things:** Do you feel powerful or happy?

8. **Slowly lengthen your spine:** Stretch up tall and expand your chest. Pull back your shoulders. Adjust and experiment a little until you feel your spine is lined up and straightened out.

9. **Extend your head up a little bit higher.**

10. **Be aware of how you feel:** What does it feel like to be upright and tall?

11. **Pay attention to your breathing:** How was it impacted by the posture change?

12. **Now say, "I am sad":** Remain in the upright posture. Does that feel strange?

13. **Learn from this experience:** Move forward in your life with this lesson. If you want to counteract shame, guilt, and anxiety, begin to carry yourself more upright and powerful.

Workbook Exercises

1. How did your body feel when you were hunched over and small? How did you feel emotionally?

2. How did your body feel when you were upright and tall? How did you feel emotionally?

Exercise 10: Tree Grounding Visualization

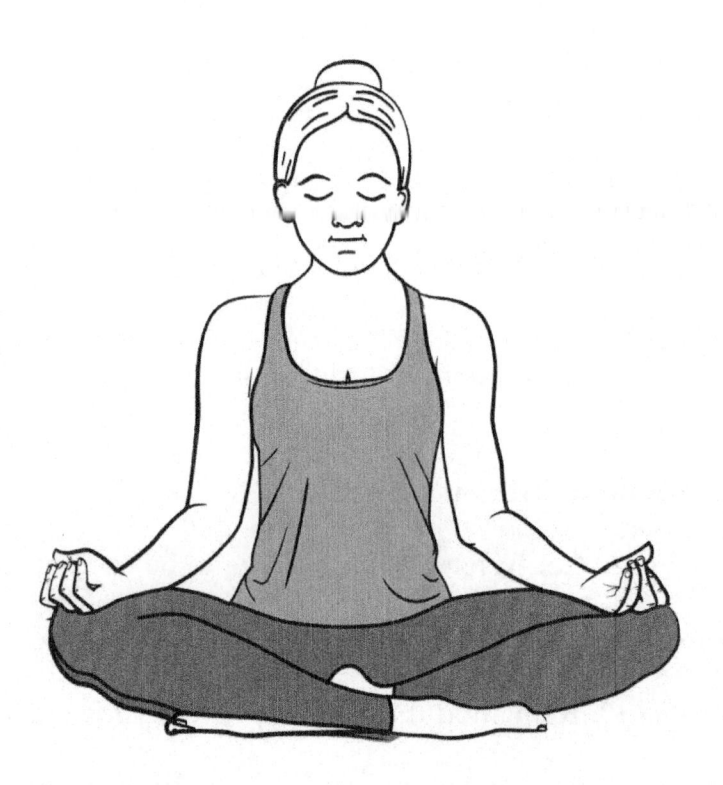

Level: Beginner

Visualization is an incredible way to supplement physical movement—or even replace it when movement is not an option. It might seem a bit complex when starting out, but its impact on the mind–body connection cannot be overstated. When you visualize, really focusing on that image in your mind, your brain can't differentiate between the image and reality. It then responds to that image as if it were really happening (Ali, 2022).

In this exercise, you will be visualizing the stalwart security of a towering tree. What do you think of when you think of a large oak? Probably strength, power, consistency. When you do this visualization, you are adopting those qualities through visualization. Let's get into it!

1. **Start by finding a comfortable place:** Ideally, this would be somewhere you can sit with your feet flat on the floor.

2. **Close your eyes:** If you are uncomfortable doing so, pick a spot and unfocus your eyes in that direction.

3. **Allow your body to relax:** Loosen your muscles, unclench your jaw, and release any tension you might have in your body.

4. **Visualize a beautiful white light coming in through the top of your head.**

5. **Imagine that light flowing downwards through your shoulders and abdomen, and down through your legs:** As it flows through you like a waterfall, imagine it loosening any remaining tension or stress that you may be holding in your body.

6. **Connect with the earth where your feet are touching the ground:** Do this by imagining the light leaving the soles of your feet and transforming into the roots of a tree going down into the earth.

7. **Allow these roots to grow thicker and deeper into the ground:** Imagine them spreading out and going through each layer of the earth, going down deeper and deeper.

8. **Sense your energy connecting closely with the energy of the earth:** You should feel strength, stability, and protection. Imagine you are one with the earth.

9. **As the roots go deeper, feel the connection to everything protected by Mother Nature:** Allow your roots to connect with the other trees and all of nature—all of Planet Earth.

10. **Sit for a moment and enjoy the feeling of deep connection, grounding, and protection.**

11. **When you are ready, open your eyes and bring your awareness back to the room.**

Workbook Exercises

1. What do you imagine when you think of a tree? How can you embody and embrace those traits day to day?

2. How did you feel before the exercise as opposed to after the exercise? Did you feel different? The same?

Exercise 11: Slight Chest Compressions

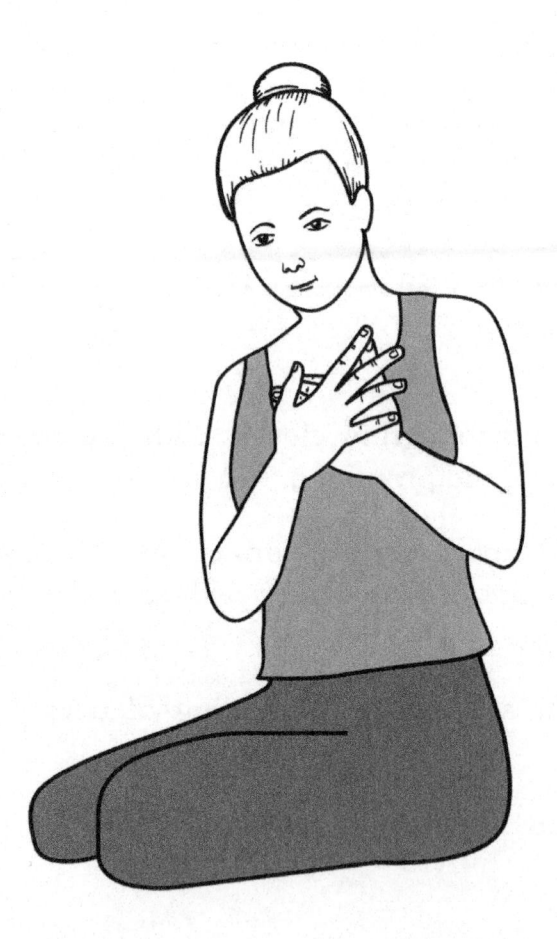

Level: Beginner

This exercise is quite possibly one of the simplest to participate in. You don't need any particular posture or location. You can be standing, sitting, or even lying down. It's less about your current moment and more about tuning into your body.

Previously, we've focused on relaxation and breathing. However, there is another body rhythm we can tune into. Our heartbeat is the very thing that keeps us alive. No matter what, as long as we are living, our heart will continue to pump blood throughout our body. Tuning into that process can give us not only peace of mind but also effective grounding.

1. **Get comfortable:** Wherever you are, get as comfortable as possible.

2. **Close your eyes and place your hand on your chest:** If you are comfortable, try using both hands.

3. **Press down on your chest with slight pressure:** Remain like this for 30 seconds.

4. **Release the pressure and rest in stillness:** Again, you want to do this for 30 seconds.

5. **Tune into your heartbeat and the breath entering and leaving your body.**

6. **Repeat several times:** Each time, check back in with yourself. How are you feeling in your body?

Workbook Exercises

1. How did you feel during the 30 seconds of pressure?

2. Was the exercise easy for you? Difficult? Explore why.

Exercise 12: Protective Force Fields

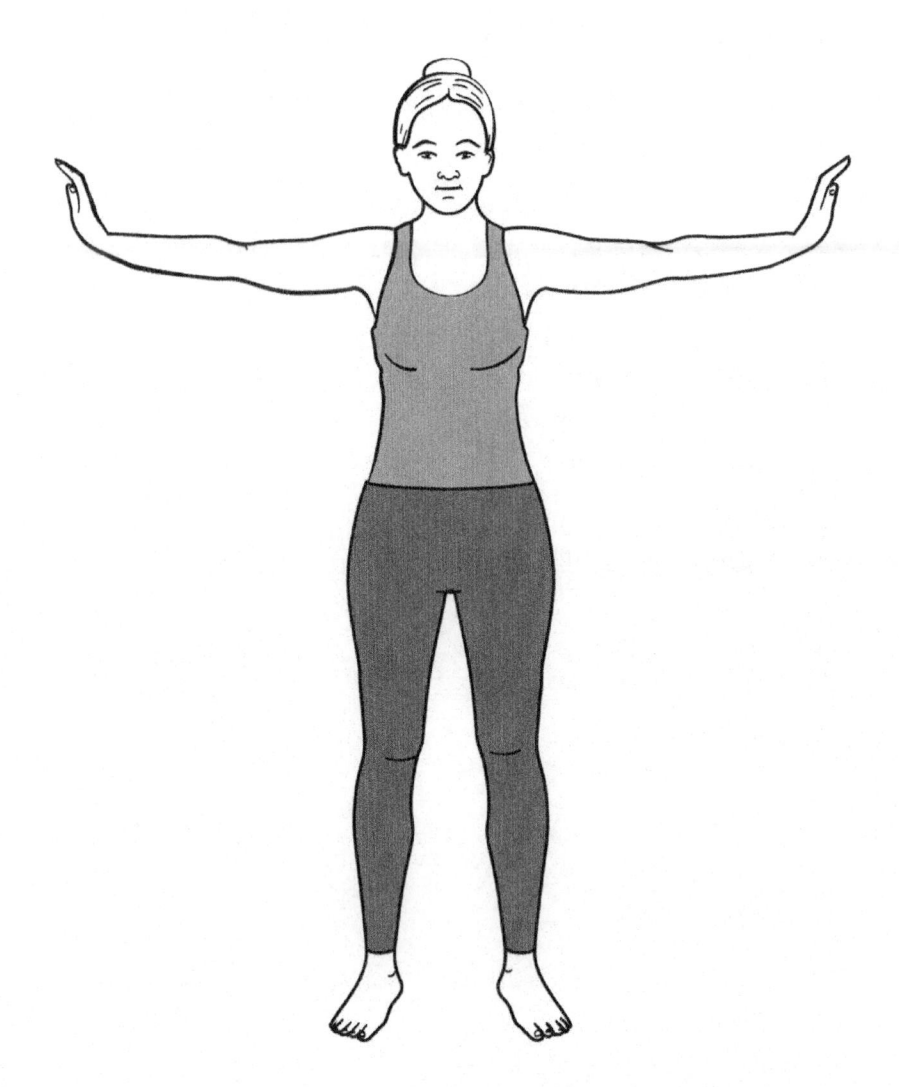

Level: Beginner

Boundaries are essential when it comes to dealing with our trauma and anxieties. At its core, trauma comes from the feeling of not being safe. So, when we protect ourselves through boundaries, we are telling our mind and body that we are safe. Safe in our environment, and safe in our bodies. Boundaries are a way of keeping harmful energy away and protecting our peace.

These boundaries are limits. They are a way of letting others know what we will and won't tolerate in our space. Whatever that looks like for you, boundaries are a great way of protecting your physical and mental well-being. In fact, studies have shown that those with healthy boundaries enjoy better overall health (Nitka, 2017).

Specifically, setting boundaries helps us avoid burnout. When we're saying yes to every request and wearing ourselves thin, we're inviting burnout into our lives. This allows for chronic stress, anxiety, and tension throughout the body. When we live with this day in and day out, the more we'll see our energy levels and immune system drop. We'll also notice a lot more aches and pains, higher blood pressure, and increased anxiety. In setting boundaries, we are protecting our physical and mental health from the impact of burnout.

In this exercise, we'll focus in on and acknowledge important boundaries.

1. **Start by imagining a big energetic bubble surrounding your body:** Be curious about the bubble. What does it look like? What is its shape?

2. **Imagine your bubble as big as you want it:** Ask yourself how much space you want and need. Imagine it growing to encompass that space.

3. **Acknowledge the size of your bubble now:** Is it bigger than it was before? Smaller? Has the shape changed?

4. **Describe your bubble:** What color or texture would you like this bubble to be?

5. **Focus on what you want your bubble to represent:** Do you want to feel protected? Comforted? Imagine and lean into that.

6. **Notice how your bubble feels in the moment:** Is it weak? Does it feel like it has holes in it, letting things slip through? Is it hard to conjure the image?

7. **Slowly reach your hands out:** Whether in front of you or to the sides, raise your arms and reach out.

8. **Move your hands and start pushing air away from your body:** You are now physically feeling the space around you.

9. **Take a look around at all the space you have in this bubble:** As you look around, keep imagining that bubble surrounding all four sides of you, up above you, and below you.

10. **Move your fingertips around the bubble:** Imagine you are painting the inside of your bubble. What colors are you using? Think of colors that conjure up fun, joy, and peace.

11. **Rest your arms when you're ready, and settle back into the image of sitting in the bubble.**

12. **Ask yourself what would you like to have in your bubble:** Maybe it's a pet or a loved one. And maybe it's just you. Maybe it's a favorite fuzzy blanket. Whatever feels comfortable. How does your body respond to what you brought in?

Note: *You might experience an activation around feeling alone in your bubble. Acknowledge and name this feeling. And perhaps imagine a doorway in the bubble. You hold the key.*

Workbook Exercises

1. What did it feel like for you to feel out your own energetic boundaries in this exercise?

2. Describe your bubble:

Breathwork

You'll notice I like to bring your attention to your breath. When this is the primary focus of the exercise, it is known as breathwork. This technique is considered something of a lost art—because it isn't new at all. Western culture has been rediscovering breathwork in recent years, but these techniques have existed in some form since ancient times.

Proper breathing starts in the nose and moves down toward your diaphragm in your lower abdomen. But the fact is, not many of us breathe this way. It is worth it to "retrain" your breathing, as there are several negative effects of breathing through the mouth, such as sleep disorders and dental abnormalities (Cleveland Clinic, n.d.-b).

By incorporating proper deep breathing into your everyday routine, you'll improve not only your mental health but your physical well-being as well. Deep breathing slows down your breathing, lowers your cortisol levels, and improves your energy levels. It can also give you a better night's sleep and calm anxiety. It is especially helpful for those with breathing conditions, such as asthma.

These exercises all focus on the act of breathwork. As you go through each technique, keep your mind and airways open. But also be mindful of any lightheadedness or chest pains, which would point to improper technique. Also, ensure that you are seated in a comfortable place while practicing these techniques. Don't attempt them while in a body of water or while driving.

Exercise 13: Voo Breathing

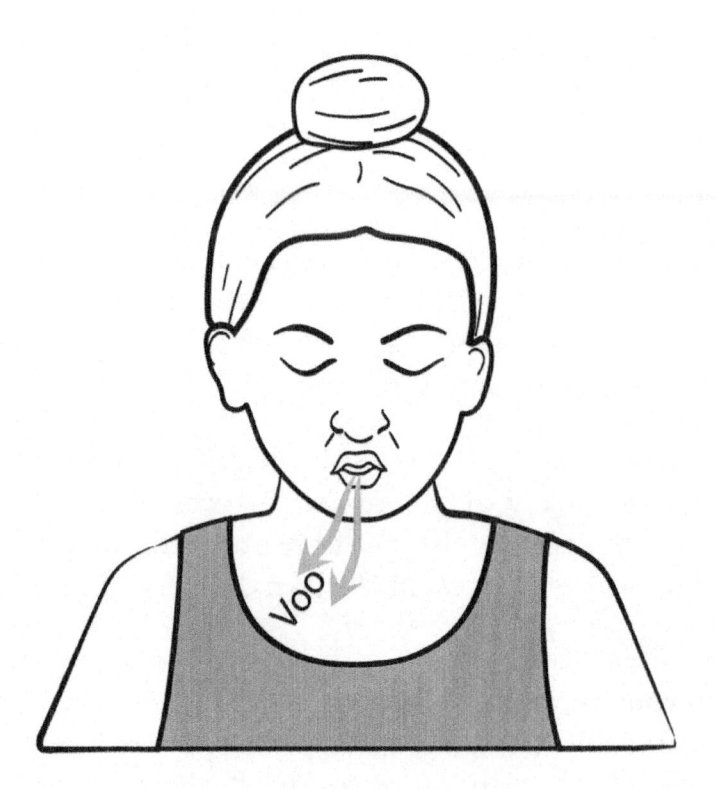

Level: Beginner

"Voo breathing" is a popular somatic technique that was developed and popularized by Peter Levine, the mind behind somatic experiencing. This technique seems simple on the surface, but it can be a deeply impactful experience when done correctly. It can calm anxiety while also giving a sense of safety. It works by triggering both the sympathetic and parasympathetic nervous systems, making the practitioner feel calm and at peace (Ally, 2020). It also activates the vagus nerve, which impacts how our body responds to stress (Keer, 2024).

1. **Start by finding a comfortable place where you can sit:** Sit upright, but make sure that there is no tension in your body. Rest your feet on the floor.

2. **Bring your focus to the feeling of your feet on the floor, and relax into the chair.**

3. **If and when you feel comfortable, close your eyes:** If you don't feel comfortable, lower and soften your gaze.

4. **Bring your attention to your breath:** Pay mind to how it enters and leaves your body. Don't try to change it just yet, but remain conscious of it.

5. **Now, take a deep breath in through your nose:** Fill your belly with the breath.

6. **Make a "voo" sound as you breathe out through your mouth:** Feel it resonate through your body. You don't need to be loud, but try to make the sound resonate throughout your body, pitching the tone low like a foghorn.

7. **When the "voo" sound ends, inhale naturally:** Breathe in slowly and naturally.

8. **Take notice of how your body is responding:** Are you feeling calmed or activated?

9. **Repeat the "voo" cycle:** Try to go for three to five minutes, remaining aware of the effect in your body.

10. **Bring your focus back to the room:** On your last exhale, open your eyes and come back to the present moment.

Workbook Exercises

1. What emotions came up for you when you did this exercise?

2. What physical sensations did you notice while doing this exercise?

Exercise 14: 4–5–6 Breathing

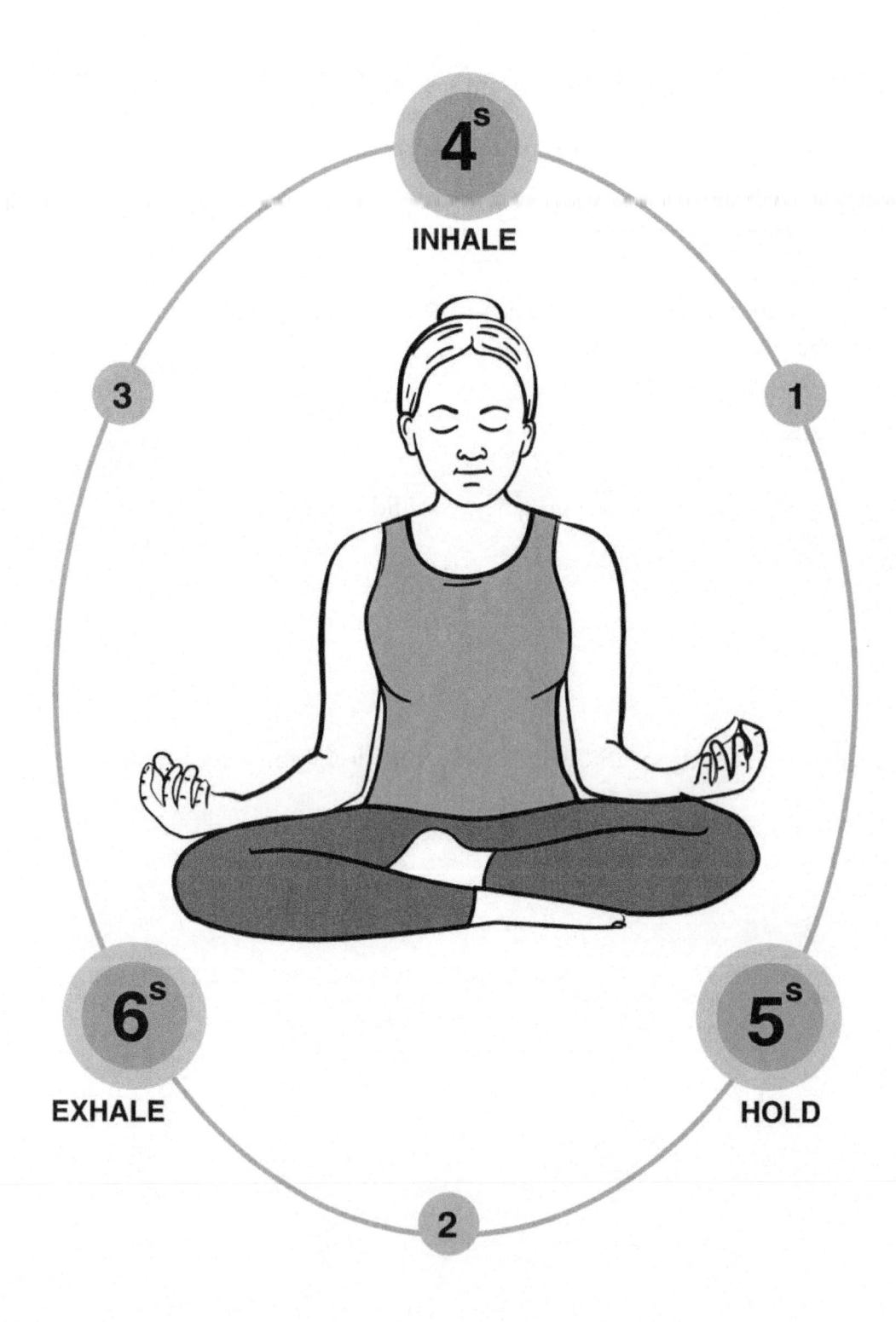

Level: Beginner

Have you ever felt incredibly overwhelmed? Maybe you're facing a big meeting at work and you don't feel ready. Or maybe it just feels like stressors are piling on, not giving you a moment to relax. In these moments, it is incredibly easy to feel dysregulated and anxious. However, we can use breathwork to bring ourselves back to center.

Breathwork, and especially the 4–5–6 exercise, has been found to increase positive emotions and balance out our heart rate. So, when your mind is racing and your heart is beating double time, this technique can help regulate you again (Fletcher, 2019). And you can do it anywhere, anytime!

1. **Start by breathing in for a count of four (4):** For those four seconds, inhale steadily through your nose.

2. **Then, hold your breath for five (5) seconds.**

3. **Finally, exhale for six (6) full seconds:** Exhale through your mouth for those six seconds.

4. **Repeat this process two to three times.**

Workbook Exercises

1. How did it feel to change and measure your breath like that?

2. How were your anxiety and feelings of overwhelm after the exercise?

Exercise 15: Pursed-Lip Breathing

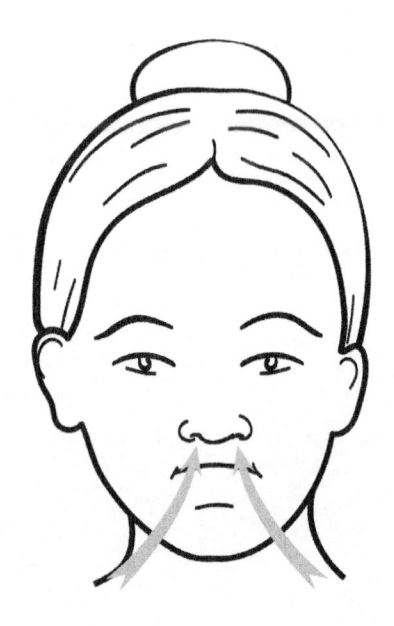

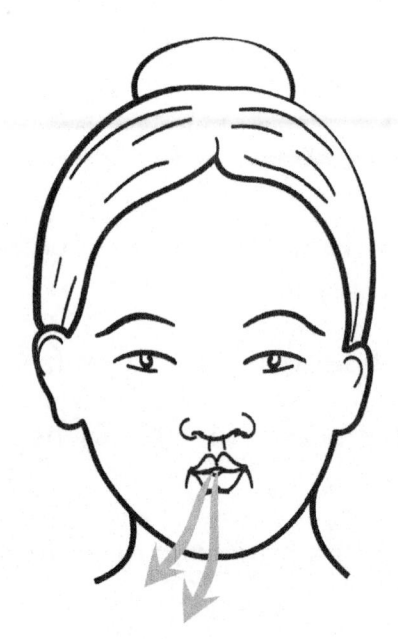

Level: Beginner

Have you ever dealt with moments of anxiety that made you feel short of breath? It's hard enough to deal with the racing thoughts and galloping heartbeat. But when you feel like it's a struggle to breathe, your anxiety can really go through the roof. Pursed-Lip Breathing is an exercise that can correct this feeling, calming any unwanted anxiety or activation.

There are many benefits to this kind of breathing. For starters, it can slow and regulate your breathing, making you feel as though you are catching your breath. It also makes the act of breathing more comfortable by clearing out the air held in your lungs. Overall, it reduces feelings of stress and anxiety (Cleveland Clinic, n.d.-c).

The exercise might feel a little awkward at first. However, as you continue to practice it, the technique will become easier and more comfortable. Just remember not to force the air out, and always breathe out for longer than you breathe in.

1. **Begin by relaxing your neck muscles and shoulder muscles:** Imagine the tension flowing out of your muscles.

2. **Inhale deeply through your nose for two full seconds:** Don't feel like you have to take a deep breath. A normal one is just fine. You should feel your stomach expand as you breathe in. If it's helpful, put your hands there to feel the movement.

3. **Breathe out through pursed lips:** Pretend you are going to whistle, or to blow on your hot chocolate in the winter. Try to exhale for about four to five seconds. If your hands are on your stomach, you should feel your stomach shrink.

Workbook Exercises

1. Did the practice feel unnatural to you at first? Why or why not?

2. What feelings came up around the practice?

Exercise 16: Diaphragmatic Breathing

Level: Beginner

I still remember when I was a kid participating in music class. To get us used to proper breathing, the teacher had us lie on the ground with our hands on our stomachs. She would tell us to feel our stomachs go up and down with each breath. This, she told us, was breathing from our diaphragm.

That was my first brush with diaphragmatic breathing. It wasn't until I got involved with somatic practices that I would understand exactly the importance of diaphragmatic breathing. Breathing from the diaphragm helps reduce the heart rate and brings on a sense of calm. But it also decreases oxygen demand, meaning it feels easier to breathe overall (Cleveland Clinic, n.d.-a).

Lying-Down Variation

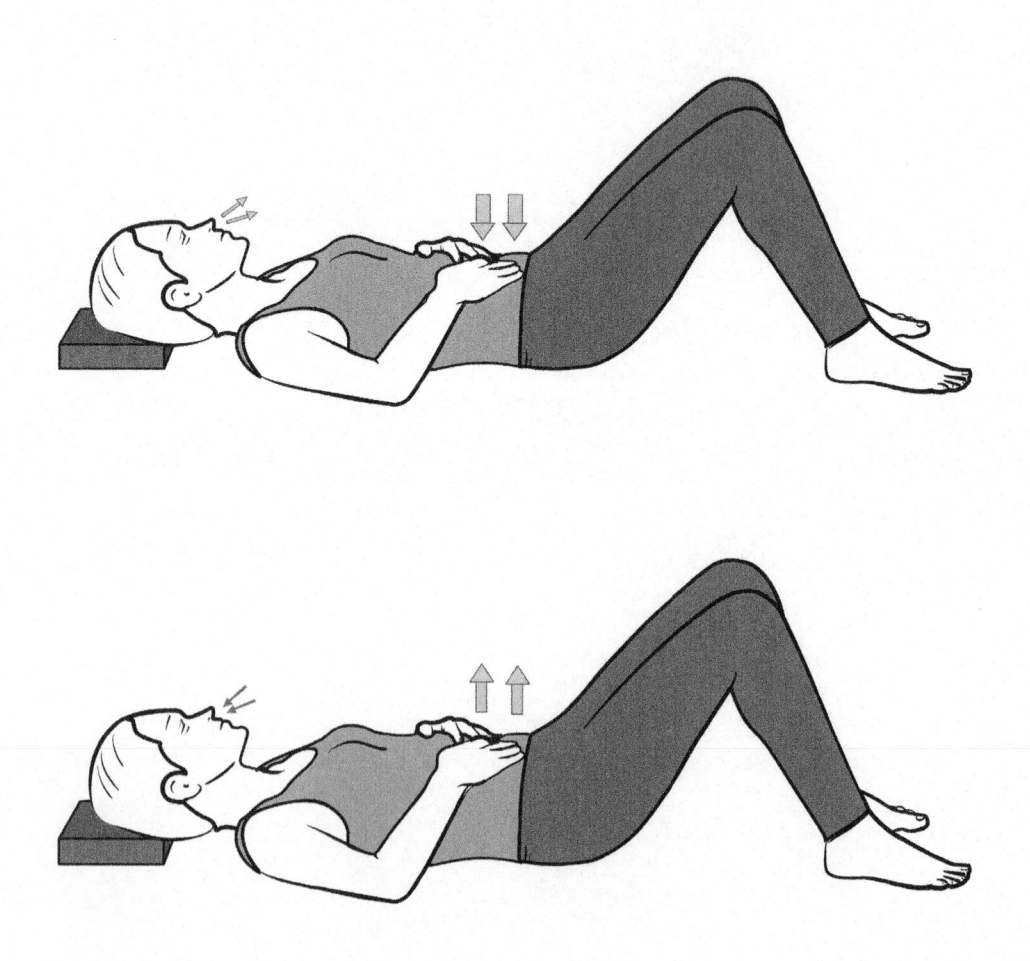

The easiest way to begin diaphragmatic breathing is by lying down, just like my music teacher recommended. This is because our body more easily defaults to diaphragmatic breathing in this position.

1. **Lie down slowly, putting your hands on top of your belly:** Ensure that you are as comfortable and relaxed as possible.

2. **Take a few deep, relaxing breaths:** As you do, notice how your breathing is reflected in your body.

3. **Now, as you breathe in, try to push your belly outward:** The breath doesn't have to be particularly deep to accomplish this.

4. **Then, as you breathe out, try to bring your belly in:** Again, this can be done whether the breath is deep or not.

5. **Repeat a few times.**

Standing Variation

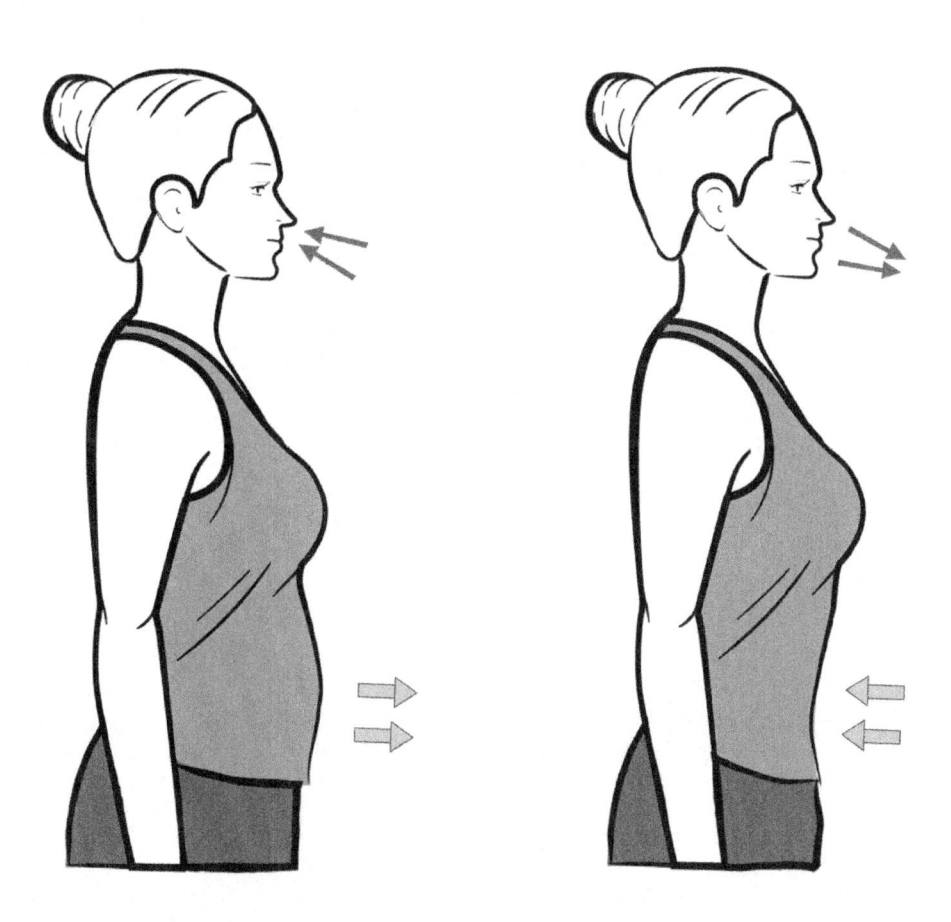

You can also do this exercise standing up. While it will take a little more intention in this position, it can often be more convenient to be standing.

1. **Stand up:** Keep your feet shoulder-width apart, knees slightly bent.

2. **Place your hands over your belly:** One hand should be over the other.

3. **Breathe in:** And as you do, try to push out your belly.

4. **Breathe out:** Now, as you breathe out, try to bring your belly back in.

5. **Repeat a few times, as needed.**

Workbook Exercises

1. Was this exercise challenging? If so, what was challenging about it? Remember, practice will make things easier over time.

2. Notice your body after this breathing exercise. What do you notice about how you feel in your body?

Exercise 17: Double Inhale Technique

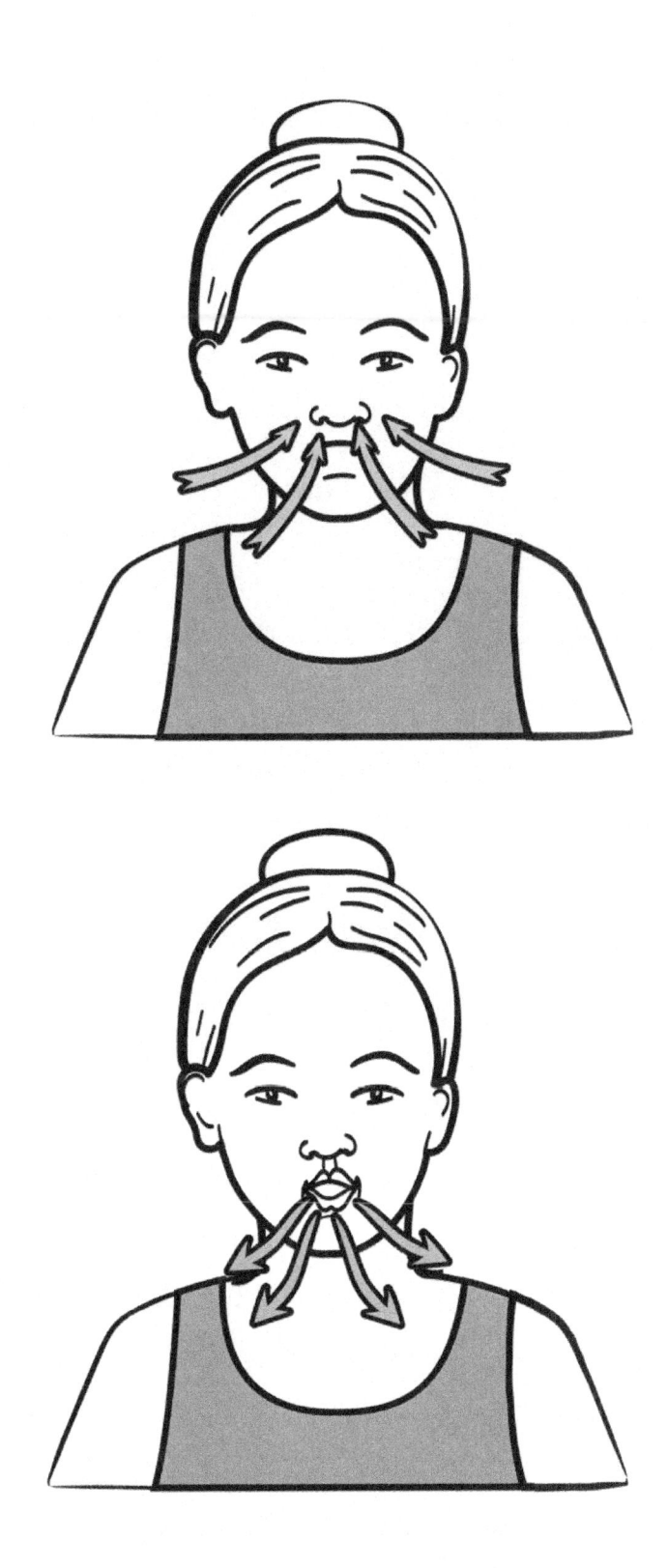

Level: Beginner

When you are feeling stressed or overwhelmed, you will often hear the phrase, "Just take a deep breath." And there's a reason for that. In times of stress, the rate of your breathing typically goes up. You begin to take small, shallow breaths. When you do this, though, the small air sacs in your lungs collapse and the level of carbon dioxide in your body goes up. Higher levels of carbon dioxide mean greater anxiety and stress (Haden, 2023). The cycle of stress perpetuates. Taking a deep breath can change that.

Sometimes, though, you need a bit of a reset button. Something to give you a jolt of oxygen and help activate the parasympathetic nervous system. Then you'll be on the right track. Enter the Double Inhale Technique. This is a great, quick way to reset the nervous system and feel immediately calmer and more balanced.

The second inhale in the Double Inhale Technique is imperative, as it helps those collapsed air sacs in your lungs reinflate. It also increases the surface area of your lungs, allowing for more efficient removal of carbon dioxide from the body (Haden, 2023).

1. **Breathe in deeply through your nose.**

2. **Pause on that inhale before taking another quick inhale through your nose:** However, if you can't inhale again through your nose for whatever reason, you can do the second inhale through the mouth instead.

3. **Let out a nice smooth exhale:** Don't force the breath out; just let it leave your body smoothly and evenly.

Workbook Exercises

1. What changed for you while doing the exercise?

2. If it's working for you, how can you implement this exercise into your daily life?

Exercise 18: Three-Dimensional Breathing

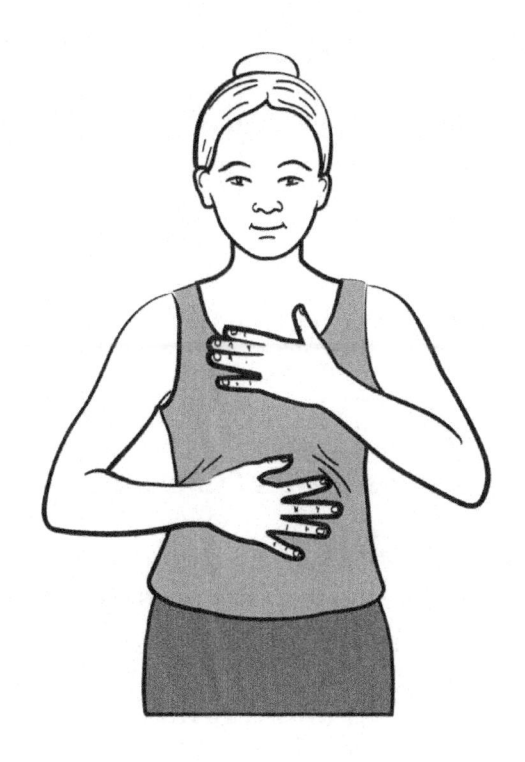

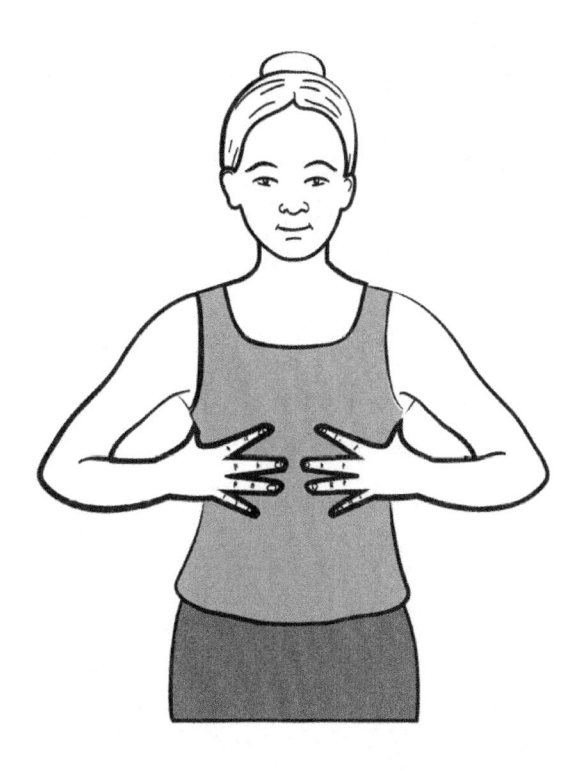

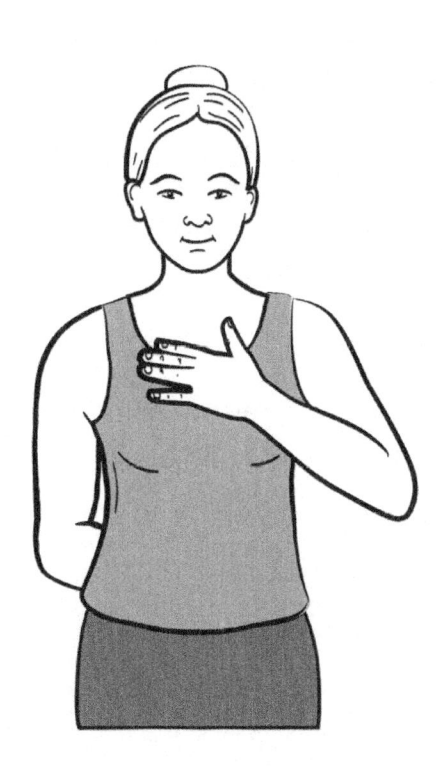

Level: Intermediate

Breathing can be described as a three-dimensional activity in your torso. From there, it radiates through the arms, legs, and head. This next exercise is meant to ensure that your lungs are expanding in all directions, fully inflating.

The truth is, most of us are actually breathing "incorrectly." I know it sounds strange to think that there is a correct way to do something that feels natural. However, breathing incorrectly can lead to everything from memory problems to higher cortisol levels (Vivos, 2022). Three-Dimensional Breathing allows us to better understand how we *should* be breathing.

1. **Put your hands on the sides of your ribs to feel the movement when you breathe:** There is a side-to-side motion to breathing that comes from the ribs opening as the lungs inflate.

2. **Next, remove your hands and *sense* that movement.**

3. **Put one hand on the top of your torso by your collarbone. Meanwhile, take your other hand and place it at the bottom of the torso at your belly:** This way, you will be able to feel the up-and-down motion in the next step.

4. **Take a breath and feel the up-and-down movement that happens when you breathe:** This is your lungs filling from top to bottom.

5. **Next, take your hands off your torso and sense the movement.**

6. **Put one hand on your chest near your sternum. The other hand should be placed on your back, flat against the spine.**

7. **Feel the breath expand your torso outward to these two points:** This is your lungs filling outward.

8. **Now, take your hands off your torso and feel the motion.**

9. **Take some time to consider what you learned from this exercise:** Did it impact how you breathe? What sensations did you notice as you breathed?

Workbook Exercises

1. What challenges did you experience when breathing this way? Remember, anything new takes practice.

2. What benefits did you notice when breathing this way?

Exercise 19: Whispered "Ah" (Rediscovering Your Voice)

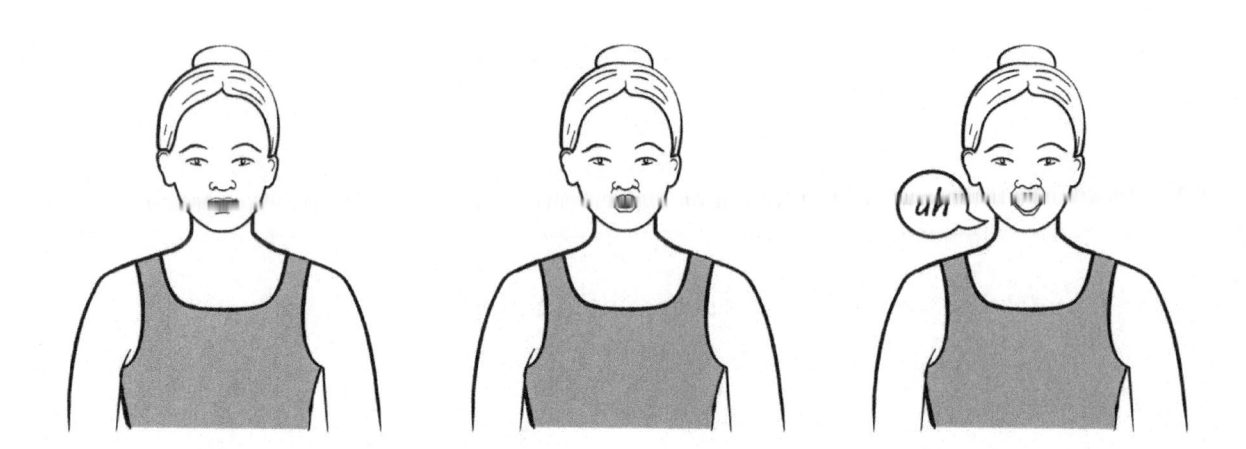

Level: Intermediate

This next exercise isn't just about breathwork. It is also about freeing up your throat, jaw, and vocal cords. The whispered "ah" doesn't just regulate your nervous system. It also causes a loosening of the jaw and vocal cords, which helps you feel more at ease in your body and your own voice. It can also alleviate the pain of TMJ disorders (Dooley, 2020).

1. **Sit with your hands in your lap:** Sit in a chair with your back straight, and lengthen your spine. Rest your hands in your lap gently.

2. **Pay attention to your posture:** You want your knees to be loose and unlocked, and gently bent. Your feet should be firmly on the ground. Allow the ground to fully support you.

3. **Think of something funny or enjoyable—and smile!** Get yourself to smile by thinking of something funny or enjoyable. This genuine smile will lift the soft palate and open up the passages of your throat.

4. **Let your tongue lie flat on the floor of your mouth:** The tip of your tongue should be touching your lower teeth.

5. **Let your jaw ease forward and drop down:** Your mouth should now be open comfortably.

6. **On your exhale, breathe out a gentle "ah" sound.**

7. **Close your mouth.**

8. **Inhale deeply through your nose:** You want this inhaled breath to fill your lungs to the top.

9. **Let your eyes be alive:** You want them to twinkle as if you were smiling at a funny joke.

10. **Again, let your jaw drop open:** Breathe out that whispered "ah" sound again, and feel it liven your system.

11. **Repeat a few times, as necessary:** How do you feel as you do so?

Workbook Exercises

1. Did any tension in your body ease while doing this exercise?

2. How different did your voice sound and feel after the exercise?

Thank you so much for making it this far!

I'm truly grateful you chose to read my book.

Among the dozens of other books you could have picked, you made the decision to take this journey with me, so a heartfelt THANK YOU for making it this far.

I want to ask you for a small favor:

If you have 60 seconds, could you share your honest review on Amazon? Posting a review is the easiest way to support the work of independent authors like myself. I always love hearing how this powerful work impacts your life!

Easy steps to leave your feedback:

1. Open the camera app on your mobile or tablet device.

2. Point your device at the QR code below.

3. The review page will show up in your web browser.

Movement Therapy

In today's world, it can be easy to fall into a sedentary lifestyle. For many, the workday happens at a desk. We are stuck in commuter traffic, seated in our car. There aren't a lot of opportunities to move our bodies. However, it is necessary for our physical *and* mental well-being that we do so. It doesn't have to mean lifting weights or running a 5k. Even gentle movements and exercises can do wonders for our health.

The importance of movement cannot be overstated. Not only does it help you manage your weight, blood sugar, and organ health, but it also helps improve your mood and calm your stress (Jagim, 2020). Meditation is powerful, but sometimes stillness is not what you need. You need to move your body to release some of that pent-up stress and anxiety.

Moving your body is especially important in somatic therapy. Movement allows us to reconnect and be comfortable in our bodies. Through different movements and exercises, you can release negative emotions and welcome in more peace and calm.

Exercise 20: Bilateral Stimulation

Level: Beginner

Bilateral stimulation refers to the presentation of alternating stimuli to both sides of the body. It is most often used in eye movement desensitization and reprocessing (EMDR) therapy, often through the utilization of flashing lights or gentle taps. During this type of therapy, the patient pays attention to the bilateral stimulation while processing difficult, traumatic memories.

However, this incredible technique can also be used in various other therapeutic endeavors. For starters, it can enhance your executive functions, improve relaxation, and reduce reactivity to stressors (Braunsdorf, 2023). With many useful applications, these related exercises will be a great tool in your therapeutic journey.

Exercise 1

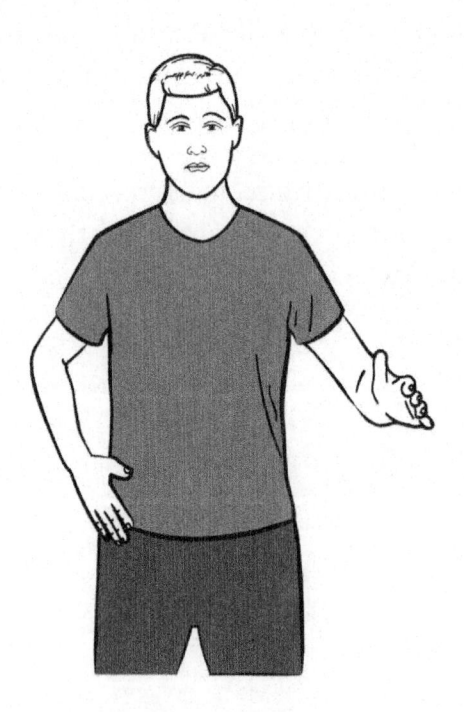

1. **Find a quiet place and get comfortable:** You can do this exercise either sitting or lying down, but ensure that you are comfortable.

2. **Close your eyes.**

3. **Take deep, purposeful breaths:** Try inhaling for five seconds, holding for a beat, and then exhaling for another five seconds. Focus on breathing from your diaphragm, and keep your breath smooth and relaxed.

4. **Recall a calming place:** Maybe it's a place where you have good, relaxing memories. Or maybe it's somewhere new but soothing, like walking through a quiet forest or sitting on a beach. Try to access all the sensory traits of the location—the crashing of the waves, the heat of the sun. Let the space fully envelop you. Do you taste anything? What do you see?

5. **Rest your hands on your legs.**

6. **Begin tapping your hands back and forth—on your thighs if sitting, or on your hips if standing:** Start with the right hand, alternating each tap from hand to hand.

7. **Tap each side about 10 times:** That is, about 20 taps overall.

8. **Notice how you are feeling:** What sensations do you notice in your body?

9. **Return to this place as needed:** Repeat this practice whenever you need to find some peace.

Exercise 2

In this exercise, we are adding in crossing our arms.

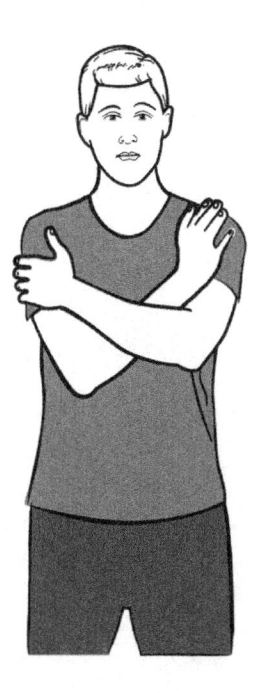

1. **Find a quiet place and get comfortable:** You can do this exercise either sitting or lying down, but ensure that you are comfortable.

2. **Close your eyes.**

3. **Take deep, purposeful breaths:** Try inhaling for five seconds, holding for a beat, and then exhaling for another five seconds. Focus on breathing from your diaphragm, and keep your breath smooth and relaxed.

4. **Recall a calming place:** Maybe it's a place where you have good, relaxing memories. Or maybe it's somewhere new but soothing, like walking through a quiet forest or sitting on a beach. Try to access all the sensory traits of the location—the crashing of the waves, the heat of the sun. Let the space fully envelop you. Do you taste anything? What do you see?

5. **Cross your arms over your chest, each hand on the opposite shoulder.**

6. **Begin tapping your hands back and forth on your shoulders:** Start with the right hand, alternating each tap from hand to hand.

7. **Tap each side about 10 times:** That is, about 20 taps overall.

8. **Notice how you are feeling:** What sensations do you notice in your body?

9. **Return to this place as needed:** Repeat this practice whenever you need to find some peace.

Exercise 3

This time, we are going to add in crossing the midline (the midsection of your body).

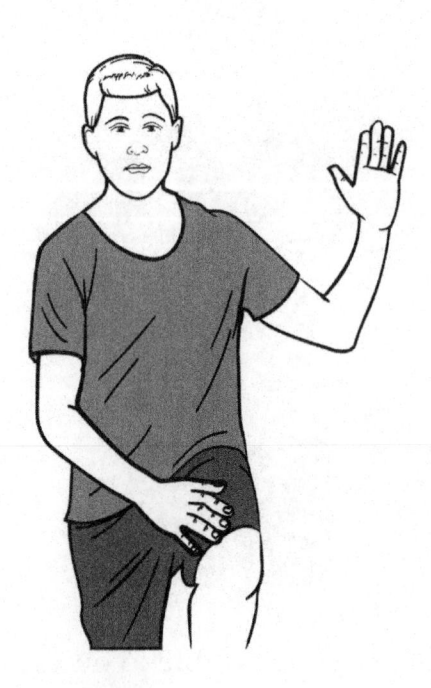

1. **Find a quiet place and get comfortable:** You can do this exercise either sitting or lying down, but ensure that you are comfortable.

2. **Close your eyes.**

3. **Take deep, purposeful breaths:** Try inhaling for five seconds, holding for a beat, and then exhaling for another five seconds. Focus on breathing from your diaphragm, and keep your breath smooth and relaxed.

4. **Recall a calming place:** Maybe it's a place where you have good, relaxing memories. Or maybe it's somewhere new but soothing, like walking through a quiet forest or sitting on a beach. Try to access all the sensory traits of the location—the crashing of the waves, the heat of the sun. Let the space fully envelop you. Do you taste anything? What do you see?

5. **Raise your right knee and tap it with your left hand.**

6. **Raise your left knee and tap it with your right hand.**

7. **Tap each side about 10 times:** That is, about 20 taps overall.

8. **Notice how you are feeling:** What sensations do you notice in your body?

9. **Return to this place as needed:** Repeat this practice whenever you need to find some peace.

Workbook Exercises

1. After the practice, notice the sensations in your body. Has anything shifted?

2. What emotions, if any, do you feel (e.g., calmer, more settled, relaxed)?

Exercise 21: Brain Tapping

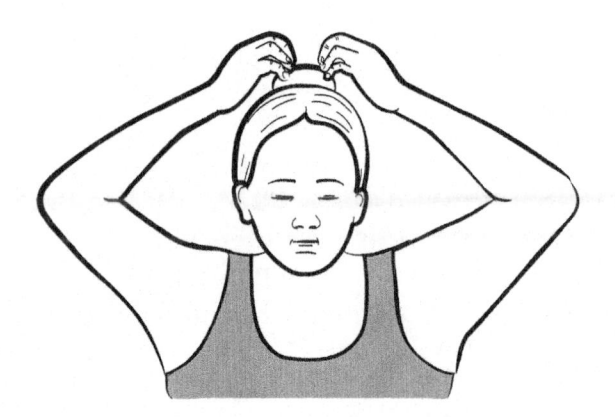

Level: Beginner

Brain tapping is a remarkable practice for those who deal with headaches. It has the ability to really clear out that blocked energy in the head, assuaging any troublesome pain there. This practice allows for better neuroplasticity. So, in addition to helping your migraines and brain fog, you are also building up resilience within the brain (König et al., 2019).

Just like the name sounds, it comes down to strategic tapping around the brain. While it sounds simple enough, the science behind it is incredible, making this a great therapeutic tool.

1. **Start in a comfortable seated position:** Ensure that your spine is straight, however. Slouching may impact the exercise's results.

2. **If you are seated in a chair, place your feet flat on the floor:** Keep them parallel, rather than pointed outward or crossed.

3. **Rest your hands on your knees and close your eyes.**

4. **Take a few deep breaths to get your mind and body in the right space to begin the work:** Breathe in deeply through your nose and out through your mouth. Do this a few times.

5. **Visualize your brain:** Keep your eyes closed as you imagine your brain floating in the middle of your head. Does your brain look healthy? Is it bright or dark? Whatever you see is okay. Just feel and observe.

6. **Slowly open your eyes.**

7. **Use your fingertips to lightly tap your brain at the top of your head:** As you tap along the outside of your skull, be intentional. Imagine the touch going through your

skin and skull, straight to your brain. Make sure you are stimulating your brain as you tap. Make sure your wrists and fingers are relaxed.

8. **Imagine lasers coming through your fingertips:** These lasers will break through any blockage in your head.

9. **If you feel pain, sigh out the pain:** Imagine it leaving your body with your exhale. The more pain you feel, the more you should exhale it out.

10. **Now, move the tapping to the back side of your head.**

11. **Now, move down to the base of your skull, tapping there as well.**

12. **Now, tap the side and back of your head.**

13. **Keep breathing out tension:** You might experience heat on your face or yawning. This is normal.

14. **Now, tap along your temples.**

15. **Tap behind your ears.**

16. **Repeat the circuit from the top of your head:** Repeat the taps along each point, tapping a little more deeply.

17. **Now, return your hands to your knees and breathe:** Feel your body with intention. What sensations do you feel after the exercise?

Workbook Exercises

1. After the exercise, notice the sensations in your body. Has anything shifted?

2. What emotions, if any, do you feel (e.g., calmness, clarity, sleepiness)?

Exercise 22: Snap–Snap–Clap Rhythm

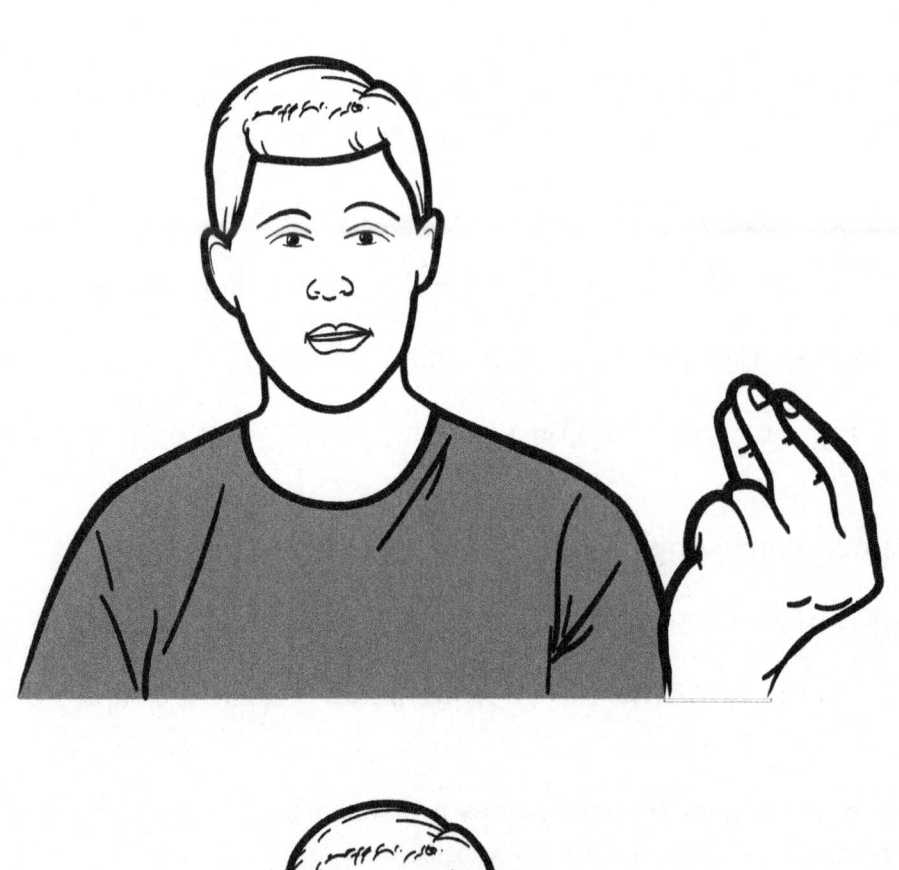

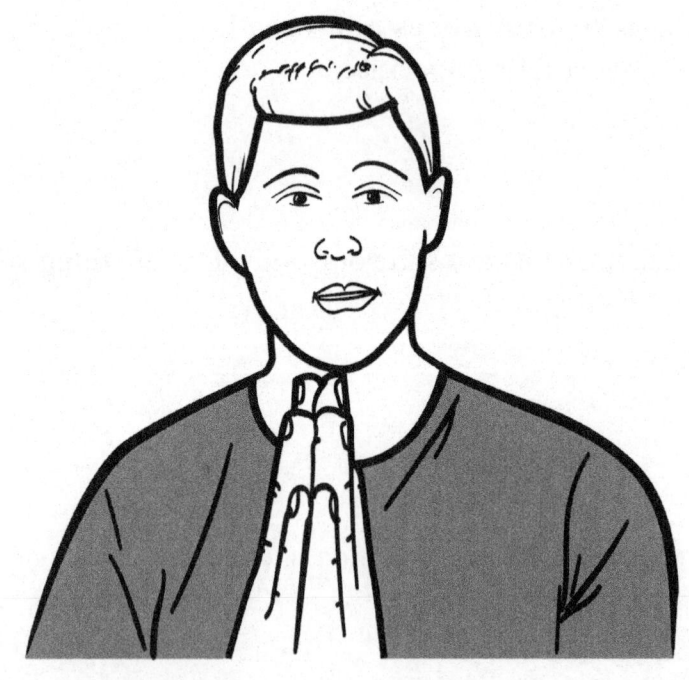

Level: Beginner

This exercise is particularly good for resetting the nervous system. That means it is great for hypervigilance, anxiety, and even chronic pain. This reset is a percussive activity and only takes about one to three minutes to practice. It's so simple and yet so profound. Even children can learn this activity and reap the benefits of the reset.

Because our brain loves patterns, this can be a soothing technique. It regulates a dysregulated system and brings us back to our baseline. It works in much the same way as bilateral stimulation does, so give it a try!

1. **Snap the fingers on your right hand.**
2. **Now, snap your fingers on your left hand.**
3. **Finally, add a clap.**
4. **(Optional) Double inhale:** At the start of the second circuit, do a quick Double Inhale (see Exercise 17).
5. **Repeat the pattern for one to three minutes.**

Workbook Exercises

1. What did you notice in your body after getting into a rhythm?

2. What variations of Snap–Snap–Clap can you add (e.g., adding a clap to the thighs)?

Exercise 23: Emotional Freedom Technique (EFT)

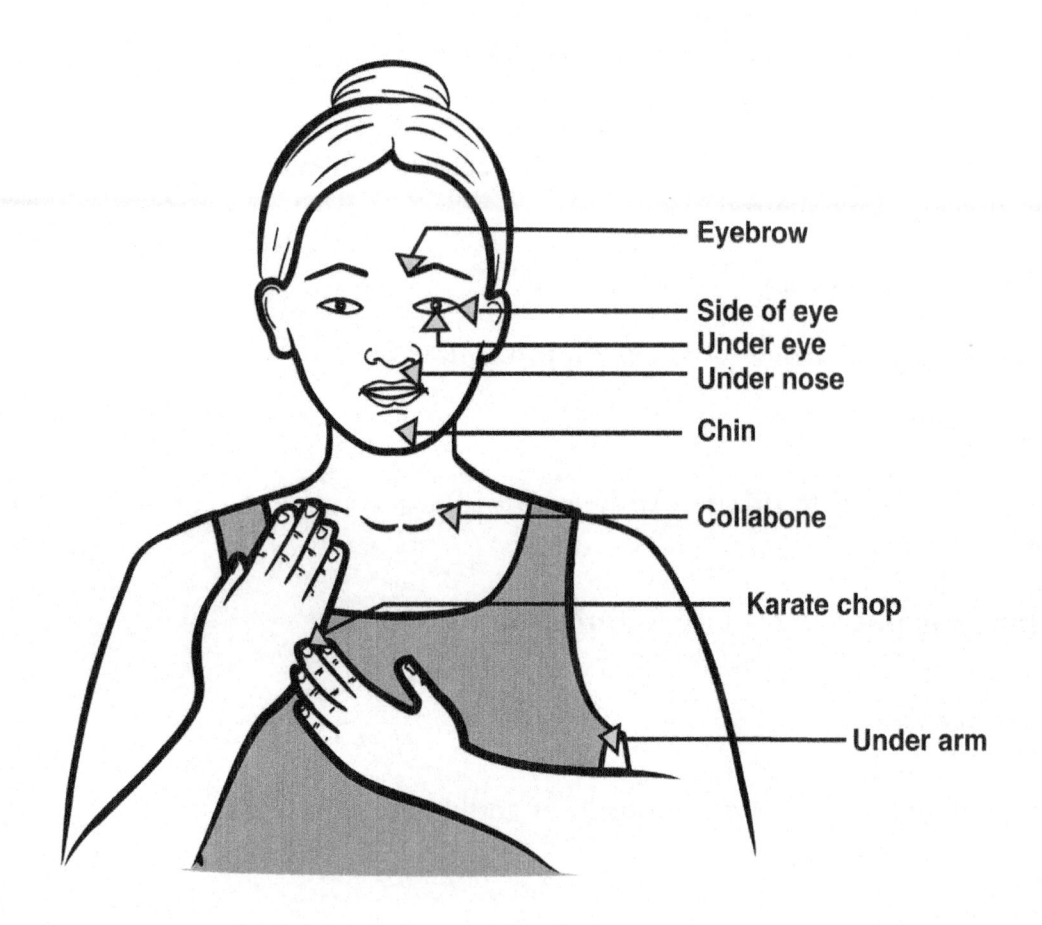

Level: Intermediate

This method utilizes rhythmic tapping on certain points of the body while you repeat key phrases. While it isn't entirely clear how this exercise works, researchers have made significant progress in identifying testable physiological and neural mechanisms. For instance, acupoint tapping calms the amygdala while decreasing physiological stress (Beer, 2024).

However, there are more benefits than just lessening stress. This technique has been shown to improve tension headaches, migraines, and even brain fog (Beer, 2024). So, if you find yourself struggling with any of these issues, give brain tapping a try.

1. **Begin by getting comfortable:** I usually recommend that someone is seated for this exercise, though it is possible to do it in any position.

2. **Identify the problem:** Be specific. Identify the discomfort or the issue you want to address. If it's a headache, feel out the pain and envision the pain being gone. This is the goal for now.

3. **Use a phrase to summarize the problem:** For a headache, it might sound like, "My head is pounding right now." Or maybe you want to focus on stress with, "Work has me feeling so overwhelmed."

4. **Rate your level of distress:** On a scale of one to ten, rate your discomfort or problem. This is entirely subjective, so go off your own scale, not someone else's. This is just a reference point for the beginning of the exercise.

5. **Create a setup statement:** Creating a setup statement includes two parts: an exposure statement that brings your problem to center stage, and an acceptance statement that recognizes the current moment as it is. For example, "Even though I feel this pain in my head, I accept that I feel this way."

6. **Repeat this phrase to yourself as you tap at the side of your hand:** With one hand, tap the outer side of your other hand as you repeat the phrase to yourself. Repeat the phrase two to three times.

7. **Repeat a "reminder phrase" as you tap other points:** A reminder phrase can be "this pain in my head" or "this headache." Tap along these points in your body:

    a. top of head

    b. between the eyebrows

    c. side of eye

    d. under eye

    e. under nose

    f. under mouth

    g. collarbone

    h. under arm

    i. back to side of hand

8. **When you have completed the sequence, re-rate your level of distress:** Has it changed at all?

Workbook Exercises

1. After the exercise, notice the sensations in your body. Has anything shifted?

   _____

   _____

2. What emotions, if any, do you feel (e.g., calmness, clarity, sleepiness)?

Exercise 24: Body Tapping (Qigong)

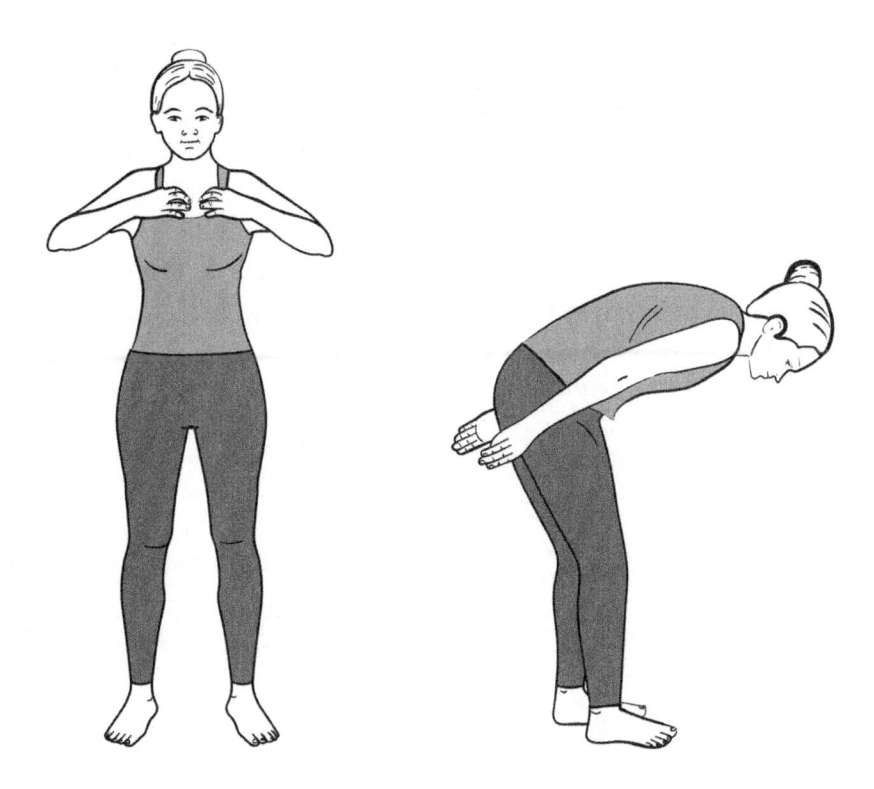

Level: Beginner

We're not done tapping! Body tapping is another name for the ancient Chinese practice of qigong. There is a lot of wisdom to be found in ancient practices. It might surprise you to realize just how connected early peoples were with their bodies. They understood the mind–body connection, and science is just now beginning to recognize their contributions to well-being.

It isn't just about mental well-being. You are also improving your immunity, neuropathy, and bone health through participation in this exercise (Jahnke et al., 2010). If you find that you often get sick, try giving this exercise a shot.

1. **Begin in a standing position with your feet right underneath your hips:** You want your stance to be shoulder-width apart. Unlock your knees. Relax into your hips. Keep your spine straight, and relax your lower back area.

2. **Relax your shoulders, allowing for a little bit of space under the armpits:** Also relax your elbows and wrists. Don't let anything lock.

3. **Bring your chin *slightly* in:** Mentally reach through the crown of the head, upwards. This will straighten and lift you up slightly.

83

4. **Activate your hands:** Begin to generate warmth by rubbing your palms together. Focus on the center of your palms first, then the fingers, and then the back of your hands.

5. **Tap along your face:** Start with the temples, moving down under the eyes and to the center of the cheeks. Then tap the top of your lip, the bottom lip, the chin, and the jaw.

6. **Rub your hands together once more:** Regenerate that heat and energy as you rub your hands together again.

7. **Tap the top of the head:** Cover the entire surface of the head—the crown, the back, and behind the ears. Start with one hand and then switch to the other.

8. **Tap the side of the neck three times:** Then tap the other side three times.

9. **Tap your upper spine:** Around the C7 area (the lowest vertebra in the neck) is best. Change hands and do a few more seconds.

10. **Body tap along your collarbone.**

11. **Tap down your arm.**

12. **Tap along the front and the back of the shoulders.**

13. **Repeat steps 10–12 with the other hand.**

14. **Tap in the chest area:** Go up along the sternum, along the lower rib.

15. **Tap along the middle back.**

16. **Move on down to the kidney area.**

17. **Tap around the tailbone:** Target the muscles around the bones to relieve any stiffness.

18. **Keep your hands cupped and tap along the top of the glutes:** Use a little more strength here. Tap all the way down the leg from here.

19. **From there, tap on the side of your legs, pause at the knees, and go down to the ankles:** Repeat.

20. **Coming down from the ribs, go down the legs:** Go all the way down to the feet and back up.

21. **Relax.**

Workbook Exercises

1. After tapping your body, what sensations did you feel (e.g., tingling, vibration, heat)?

2. After you'd tapped your body, how did you feel (e.g., relaxed, energized, relieved)?

Exercise 25: Eye Movement Routine (Qigong)

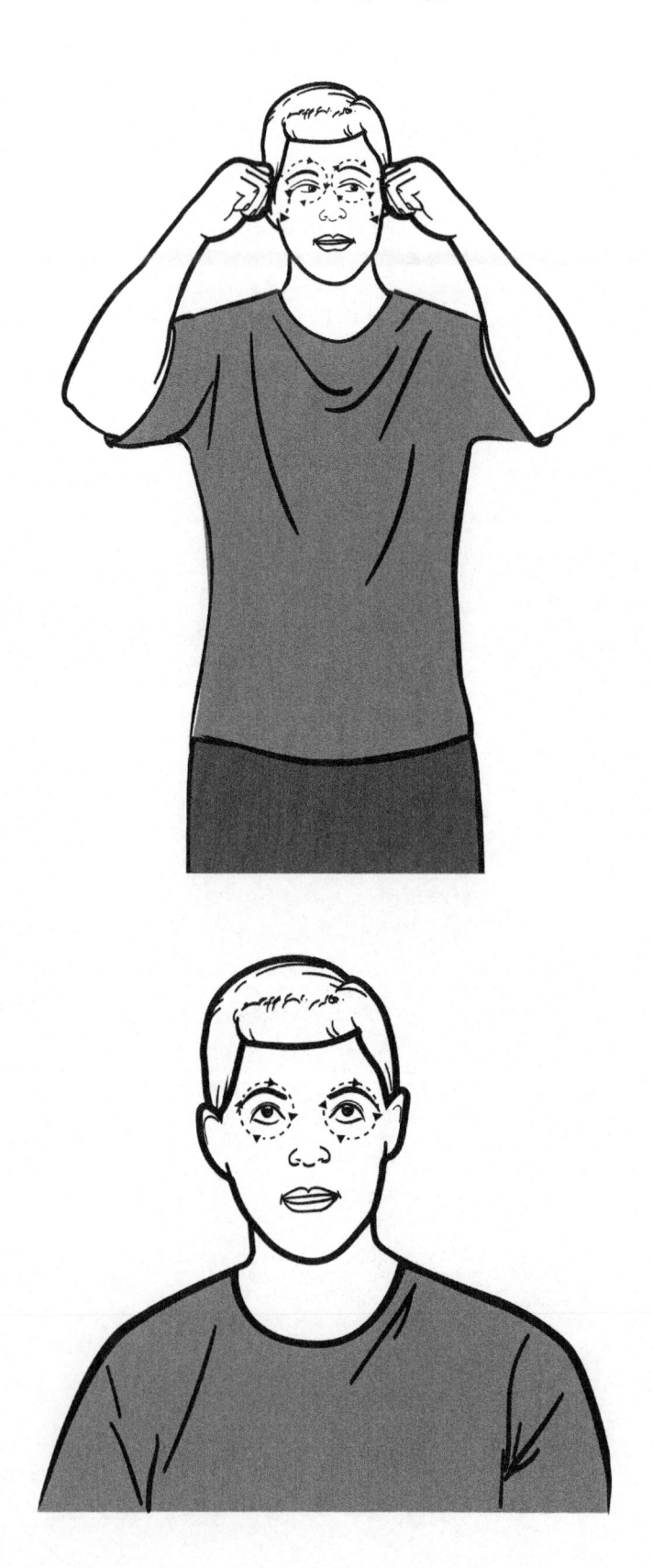

Level: Beginner

In this exercise, we return to qigong for something a little different. Rather than tapping, this technique utilizes movement of the eyes. This practice is particularly useful for anyone who spends a lot of time on the computer day to day. Staring at a screen for any length of time can cause eye strain and even pain in the eyes. Exercises like these are there to help relax those eye muscles.

This technique, and others like it, are incredibly useful when fighting against macular degeneration. That's right—these exercises don't just help you with strain, but can even prevent loss of vision (Hilal et al., 2022).

1. **Fold your first knuckle in on both hands:** Use those knuckles to rub right across the eyebrows.

2. **At the temples, make little circles with your knuckles.**

3. **Also make circles below the eyes.**

4. **Repeat a few times.**

5. **Now, drop your hands and make big circles with your eyes:** Look up, to the right, down, and to the left. Make those big circles. This strengthens the muscles.

6. **Notice where and how it is difficult to move your eyes in certain areas.**

7. **Take a deep breath:** And relax.

Workbook Exercises

1. Before the exercise, my eyes felt:

2. After the exercise, my eyes felt:

Exercise 26: Swaying Bamboo (Qigong)

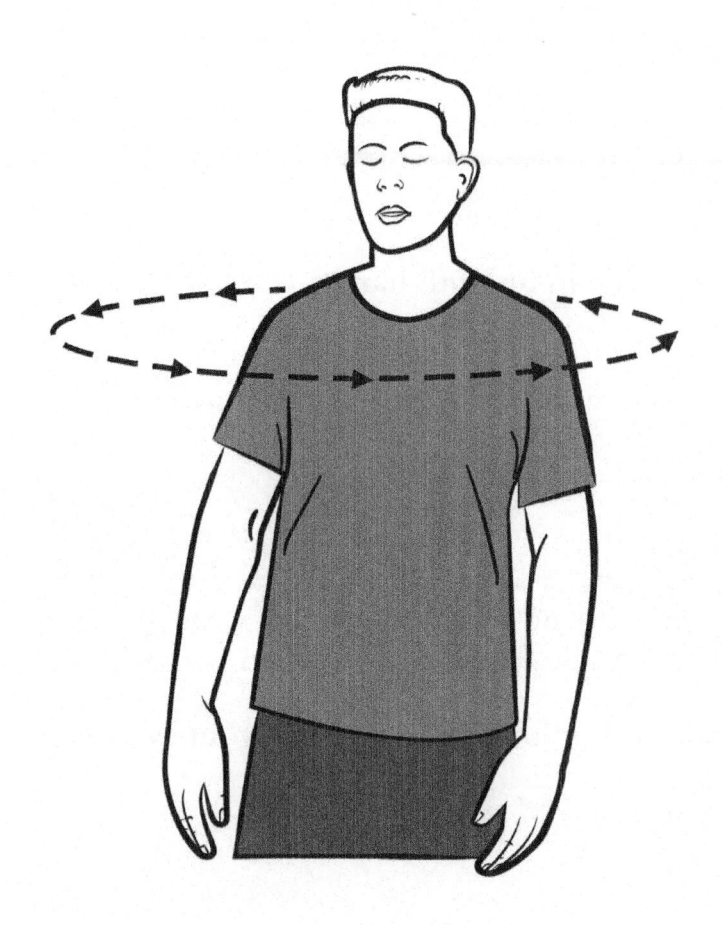

Level: Beginner

This is yet another exercise that draws from qigong, and is known as Swaying Bamboo. The exercises under the qigong umbrella emphasize the whole body, drawing from the energy within. This particular exercise brings our attention to a rocking—or swaying—motion to bring a soothing feeling to our body.

It's scientifically backed, too! The gentle horizontal rocking or swaying motion has been shown to promote better relaxation and sleep. This might be, in part, because the motion mimics the motion of being in the womb, our first natural state (Schwede, 2024).

1. **Begin in a standing position, with your hands over your belly:** Lengthen your spine and unlock your knees, settling into your legs gently.

2. **Close or unfocus your eyes:** Whatever is more comfortable for you.

3. **Begin to notice the natural sway of your body.**

4. **Allow your body to follow this natural swaying motion:** Don't force the motion; instead, just allow it to happen.

5. **Take a few deep breaths as you sway:** In through the nose, out through the mouth. Let your back be open and loose as you sway.

6. **Picture a piece of bamboo swaying in the wind as you rock from side to side:** Sink into this image as you breathe through the motions. Let your mind unwind and relax.

7. **When you are ready, bring your attention back to the present moment:** You can open or focus your eyes, then end the swaying motion when it feels right to you.

Workbook Exercises

1. Before the swaying, my body felt:

2. After the swaying, my body felt:

Exercise 27: Shaking (Qigong)

Level: Beginner

It might sound a little silly, but Taylor Swift was onto something with her hit song "Shake It Off." Researchers have actually observed that this practice comes straight from nature. Animals, from deer to dogs, will actually "shake off" tension and stress (Vinall, 2021). And it might be helpful for us to take a page out of their book.

"Shaking it off" can combat both acute and chronic stress. Shaking the body can release tension and trauma, allowing for better regulation of the autonomic nervous system, which means better regulation of our automatic bodily functions. So, digestion, heart rate, metabolism, and blood pressure are all positively impacted when you participate in this simple exercise (Vinall, 2021). You'll also see a decrease in anxiety and depression, as well as a reduced risk of things like diabetes and obesity.

This is likely because shaking can burn off extra adrenaline and relieve tension. All of this returns you to a more neutral state, which is what you can use this exercise for—returning yourself to center.

Standing Variation

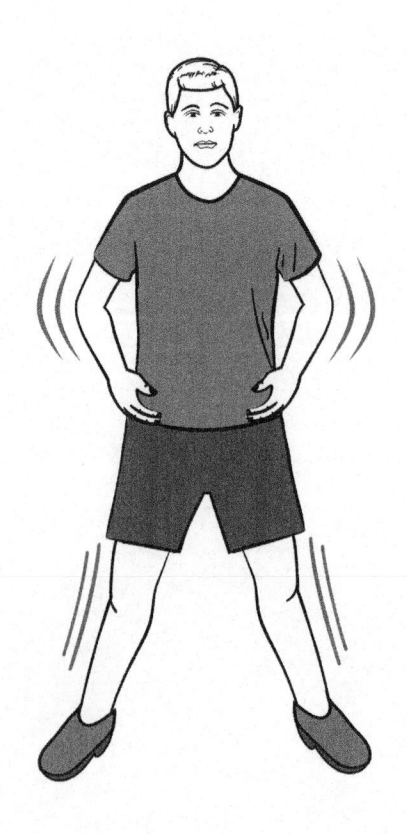

1. **Stand with your feet shoulder-width apart:** Keep the knees soft and unlocked.

2. **Relax your arms, elbows, and wrists.**

3. **Start bouncing your knees:** The knees should be like springs as you gently bounce.

4. **Breathe deeply into your belly:** As always, inhale through the nose and out through the mouth.

5. **Imagine that your center is just bouncing up and down gently like a rubber ball:** This will keep you on the right track with your movement.

6. **Your arms are loose, and should be gently swaying and shaking as you go up and down:** Don't force the motion; just let the arms shake and sway as you bounce along.

7. **Try to make an audible sigh on your exhale as you shake:** This will help you release more tension as you go.

8. **Imagine your body loosening as you continue to shake:** The legs loosen, as do the pelvis and the lower and upper spine, all the way to the neck and head. Don't control any of the movements; rather, just allow them to happen.

9. **Three or five minutes of shaking should be sufficient.**

10. **Relax your body.**

Lying-Down Variation

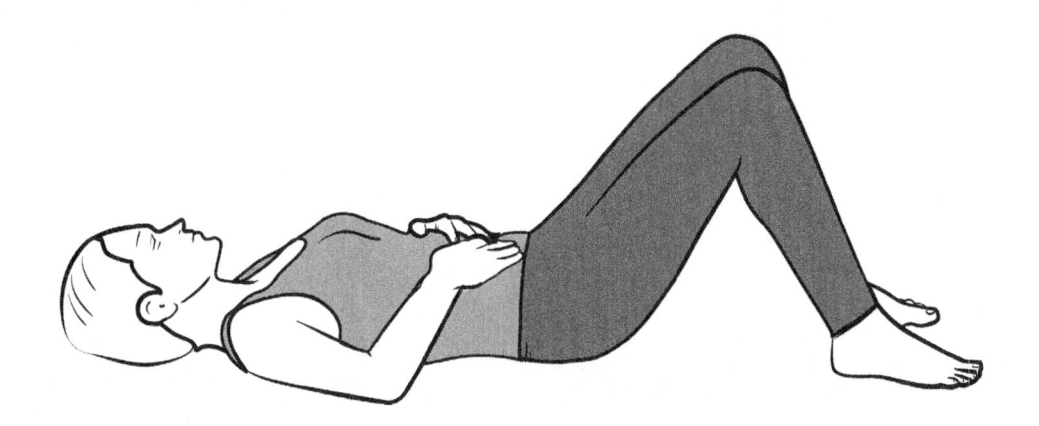

1. **Lie down comfortably on the floor:** Have your feet flat on the ground and your knees pointed up toward the ceiling.

2. **If you have any shaky or uncomfortable feelings, imagine them leaving through your feet:** They are seeping out of the soles of your feet and into the earth.

3. **Gently press into your feet:** In doing so, create a rocking sensation throughout the body. This will look different for each person. Don't overthink it, and keep your breaths natural.

4. **Continue for three to five minutes.**

5. **Relax your body.**

Workbook Exercises

1. Which parts of your body felt shaky? Which parts felt most alive?

2. After the exercise, recognize how your body feels now. Describe the difference.

Exercise 28: Opening (Qigong)

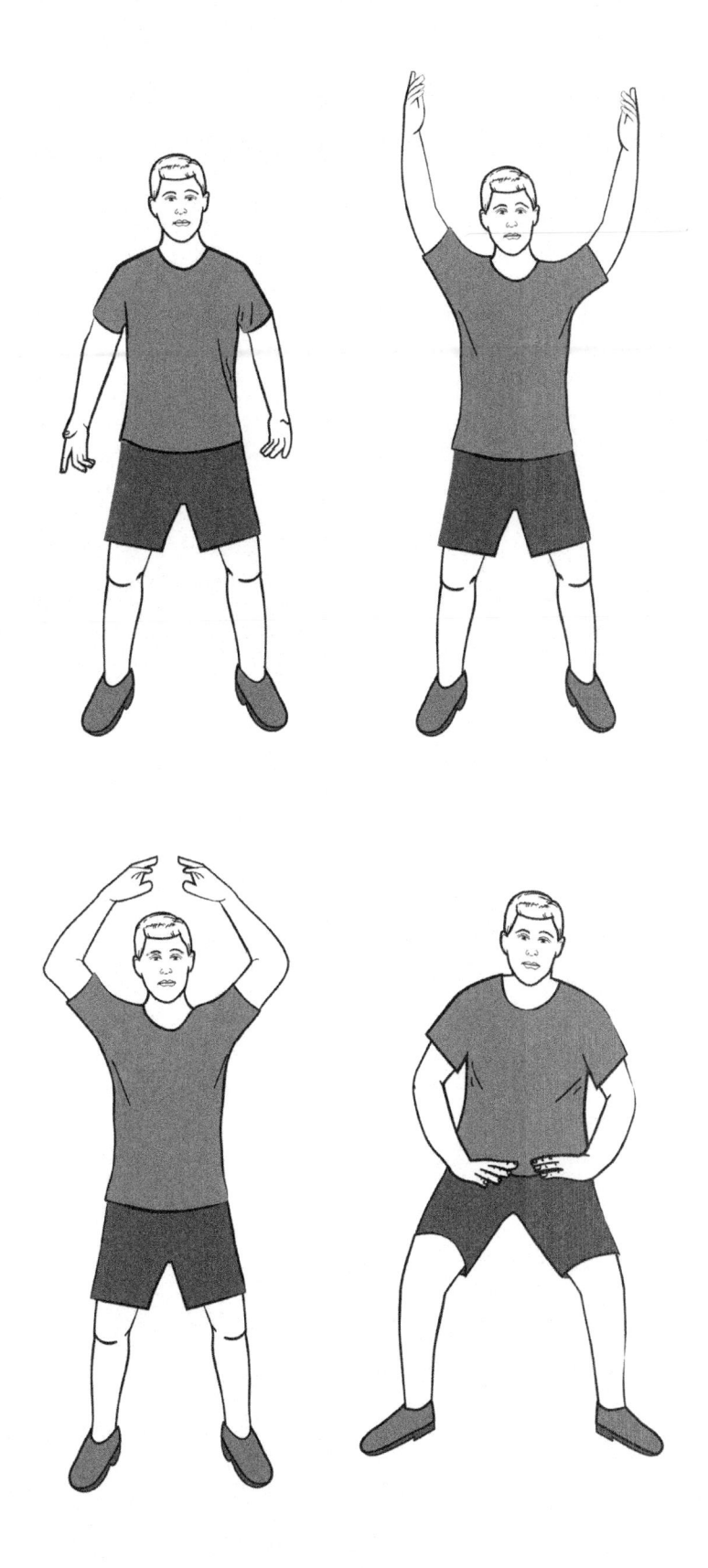

Level: Beginner

This qigong exercise is very practical and simple. You can practice it anywhere as the need arises, and there are incredible benefits. As you move the qi through the body, you are allowing for better immunity, better sleep, less stress, and a better mood (National Center for Complementary and Integrative Health, 2022). You are also allowing for better organ health. You achieve this through fluid, easy movements like the ones in this exercise.

1. **Stand very comfortably:** Unlock your knees and rest into your legs. Relax your palms at your sides.

2. **As you breathe in, your hands should come up and around:** They should nearly meet above your head, palms facing each other.

3. **As you breathe out, your hands should come down to your center:** As the breath ends, your hands should be around hip level, wrists bent toward you and knees bent.

4. **Repeat:** Bring your hands back up with the inhale, and back down to center with the exhale.

5. **Do this a few times:** As your body begins to relax, focus on your breaths in and out through the nose.

Workbook Exercises

1. As you breathed along with the motions, what did you notice in your body?

2. How do you feel now, after the exercise?

Exercise 29: Lifting the Ball (Qigong)

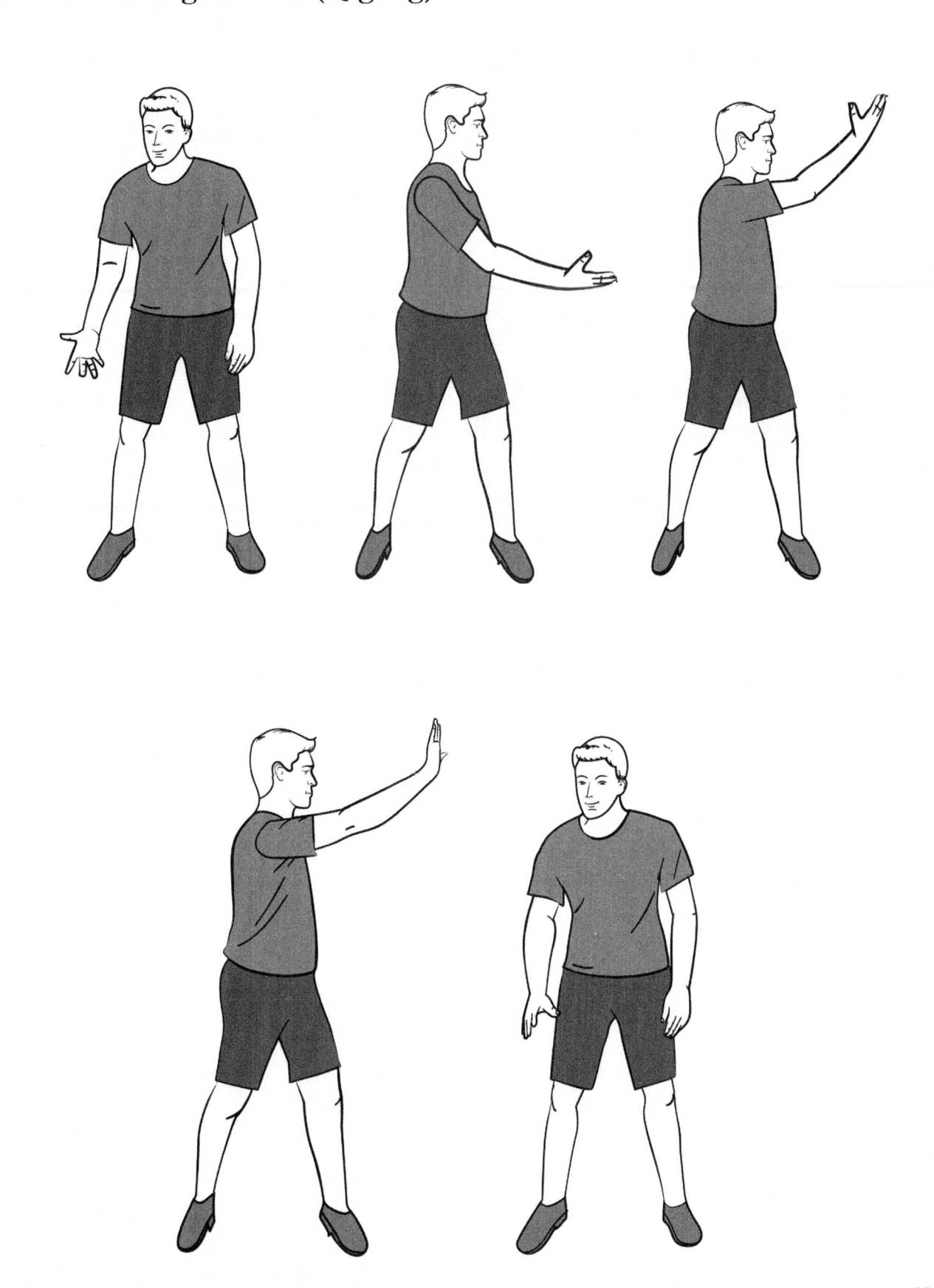

Level: Beginner

This qigong exercise is also known as *Shibashi* and benefits the kidneys as well as the flexibility of the spine. Something I particularly enjoy about this exercise is that it encourages a nature of playfulness and joy. It is said to help us embrace the feeling of freedom and childlike wonder that we are often missing.

1. **Begin by standing naturally:** Stand comfortably and naturally, while keeping the spine somewhat lengthened and straight.

2. **Turn your palms upward at your sides:** It should feel as though you are cupping something in your palms.

3. **Inhale as you turn to the left, lifting your right palm toward your left shoulder as you do:** You want your palm to end up a little above your right shoulder.

4. **Move your weight to your left leg and stretch your right leg onto your tiptoe:** This is optional, but if you would like to do so, you can lift the toes of your right leg and softly tap the ground.

5. **On your exhale, move back to center.**

6. **Immediately shift your weight to your right leg.**

7. **Now, mirror these steps on the opposite side.**

8. **Repeat six times:** As you do, focus on how the body and breath work together through the movements.

Workbook Exercises

1. How did it feel to move with your breath? Was it easy? Difficult?

2. How did you feel after the exercise?

Exercise 30: Frolicking in Water (Qigong)

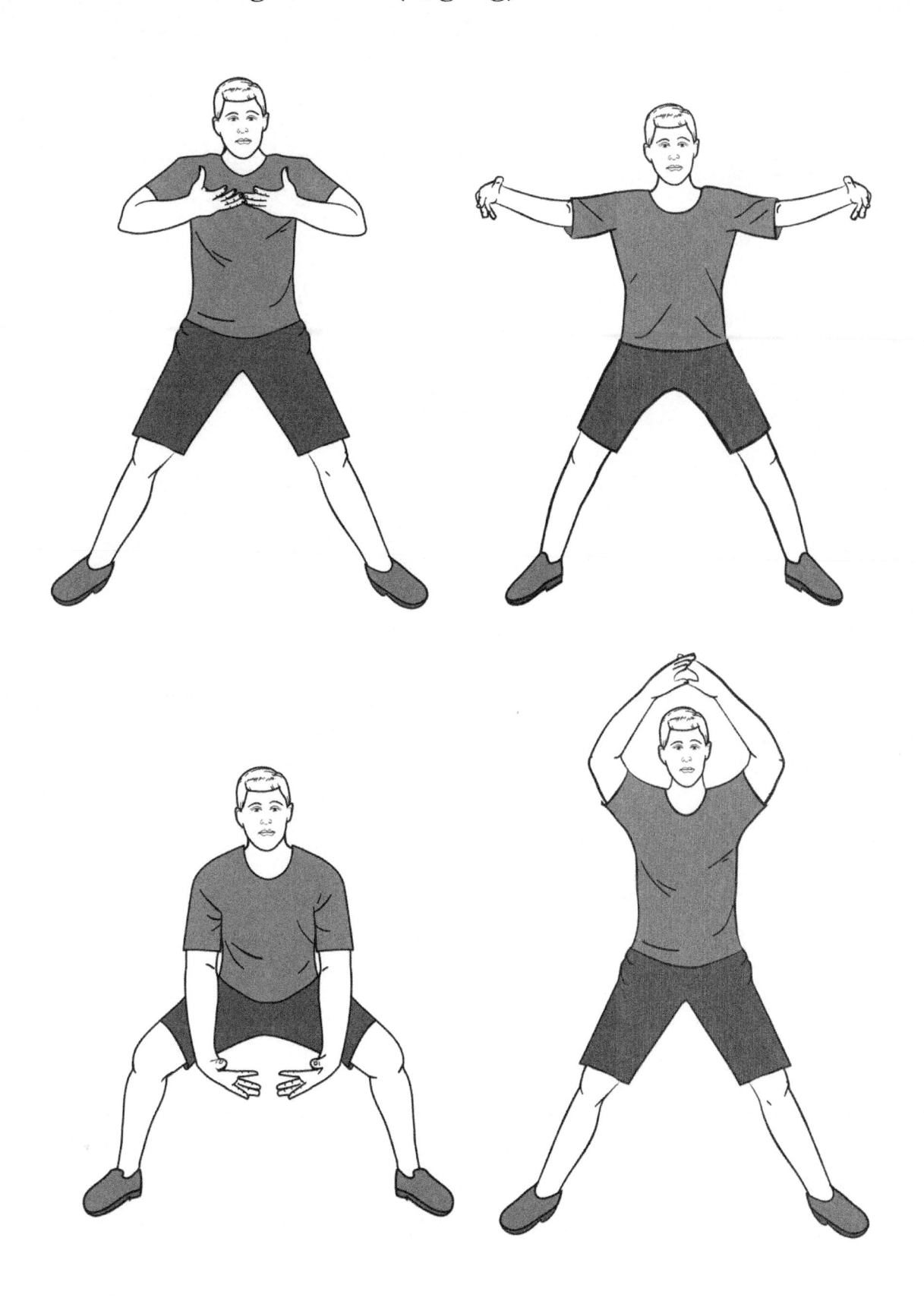

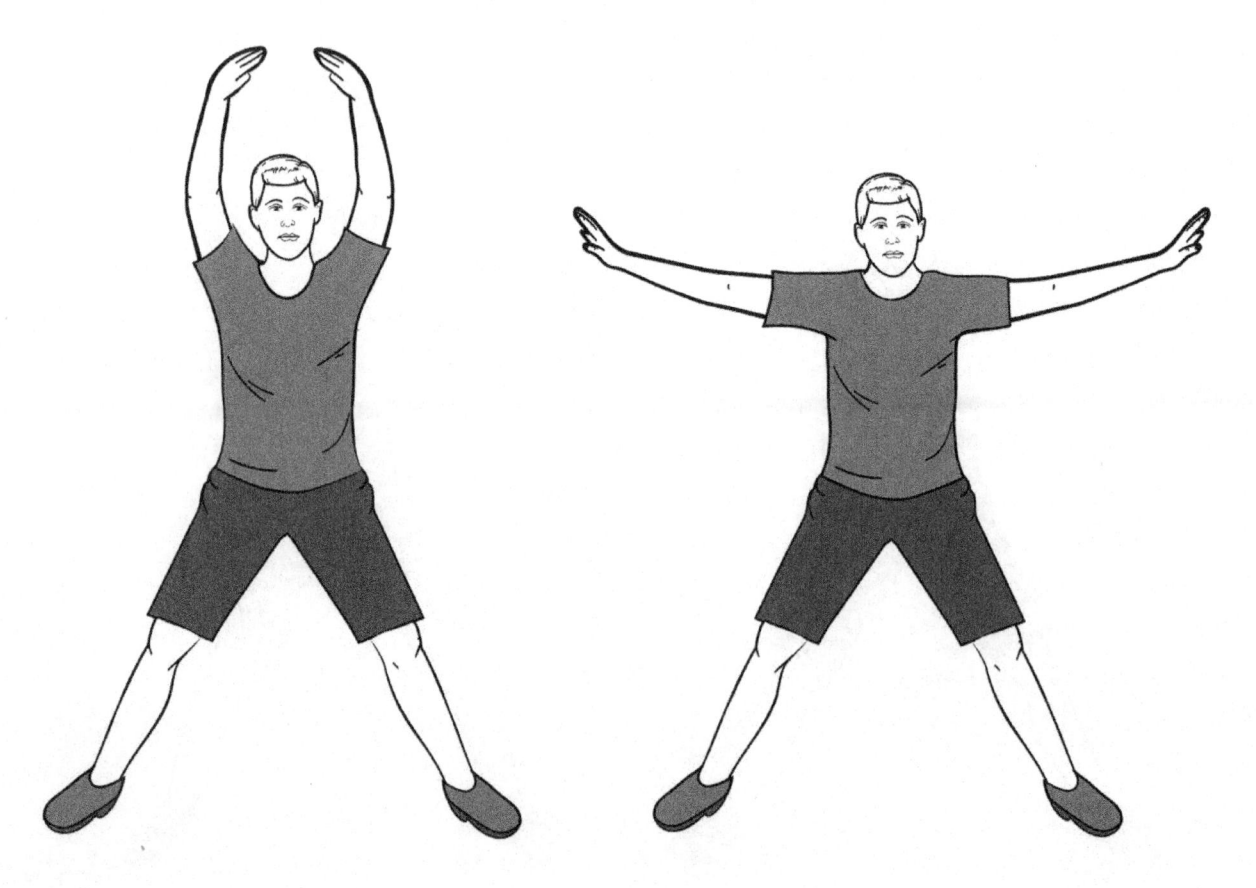

Level: Beginner

As we wrap up the qigong exercises with Frolicking in Water, I want to make note of something: You can combine all of these exercises to create a "flow." This is basically a qigong routine that works together. Combining these activities can have incredible benefits, so consider making a flow that fits well into your everyday routine.

A lot like the last exercise, this exercise can help you embrace a lighter, happier mood. It is playful and taps into that easy joy you get from moving your body.

1. **Stand with a wide stance:** You want your feet to be further than shoulder-width apart for this exercise.

2. **Start with your arms stretched outward at shoulder level:** Now, scoop downward toward your pelvis, like you are scooping up water. Inhale as you do so.

3. **Bring your hands up together, up through the center:** Come all the way up and "throw" the water out to the sides, palms facing away from you. You want to go all the way up above your head. Exhale as you do so.

4. **Repeat this motion several times:** It should be a somewhat circular movement to your sides.

5. **Let go of any tension as you repeat these motions.**

Workbook Exercises

1. How did it feel to go through these motions? Did any emotions or feelings come up for you?

2. How did you feel after the exercise (e.g., more relaxed, lightheaded, etc.)?

Exercise 31: Lizard Walk

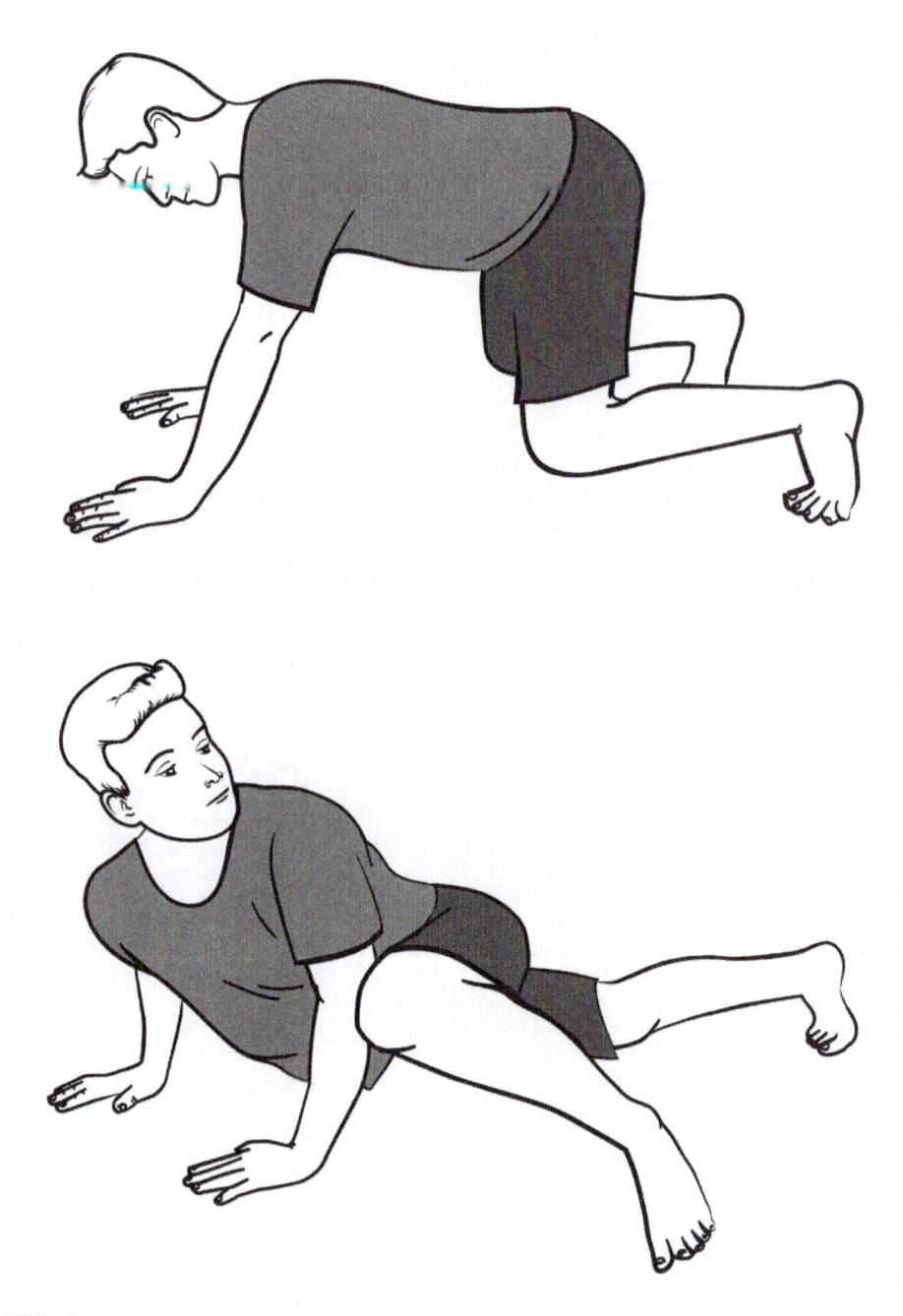

Level: Intermediate

The Lizard Walk is a great way to step into our more intermediate exercises. Not just a wonderful exercise for somatic therapy, this technique has also been adopted by fitness gurus, as it helps work certain muscle areas like the core muscles and the deltoids. Alongside exercising your muscles, it's extremely beneficial for balance and joint health (Tsong, 2023).

Precautions

However, it's important that you are safe when performing this exercise. This can be more strenuous than some of the other exercises in this book and therefore should be tackled with care. If you have any wrist, hip, back, or knee injuries, it's best to avoid this practice for now. Wait until you are healed, and then ease into exercises like this. You want to ensure you are listening to your body.

1. **Get on your hands and feet, with your knees bent toward the ground**

2. **Bring the left foot forward while bringing the right hand forward at the same time:** Look toward the left, and lean into that motion.

3. **Notice your body's alignment:** See how one leg is bent to the side so the hips are more open.

4. **Shift the weight to the opposite side.**

5. **Repeat with the opposite side.**

6. **Don't force the motion, but allow your body to move fluidly:** This movement can feel unusual at first, and it might take time for your body to adapt.

7. **Do a few sets of these movements.**

Workbook Exercises

1. After the exercise, bring your awareness to your spine. Do you notice that anything has shifted?

2. Now, bring your awareness to your hips. How do they feel?

Releasing Tension

Why is releasing tension so important to our mental well-being? We often don't question the impact tension has on our physical health. We can feel it. When we're tensed up, our muscles get tired and sore. We get headaches. We might even get stomachaches! But there is also a clear mental connection. When we have a tense body, we often have a tense mind. And vice versa! Being able to release that tension can put us in better physical and mental health.

When you are commuting to work during crazy traffic, preparing for a meeting, or running late for an appointment, you're stressed. You're tense. And your body reacts by tensing up your muscles and tendons. The next thing you know, you're stressed *and* you're dealing with pain. The way to fix that? Releasing the tension.

The next few exercises are going to be focused on releasing that tension. As you take part in these exercises, imagine the tension leaving your body in waves. Visualization can often be a factor in how we release tension, so adding components like this can be beneficial.

Exercise 32: Softening the Gaze

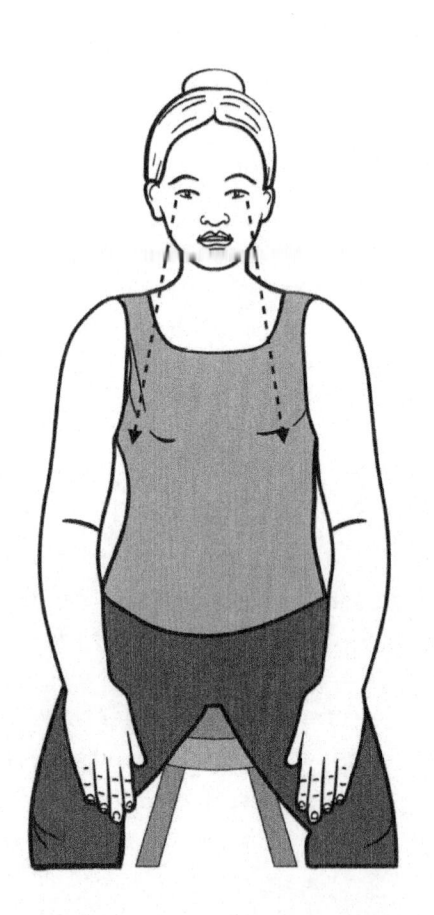

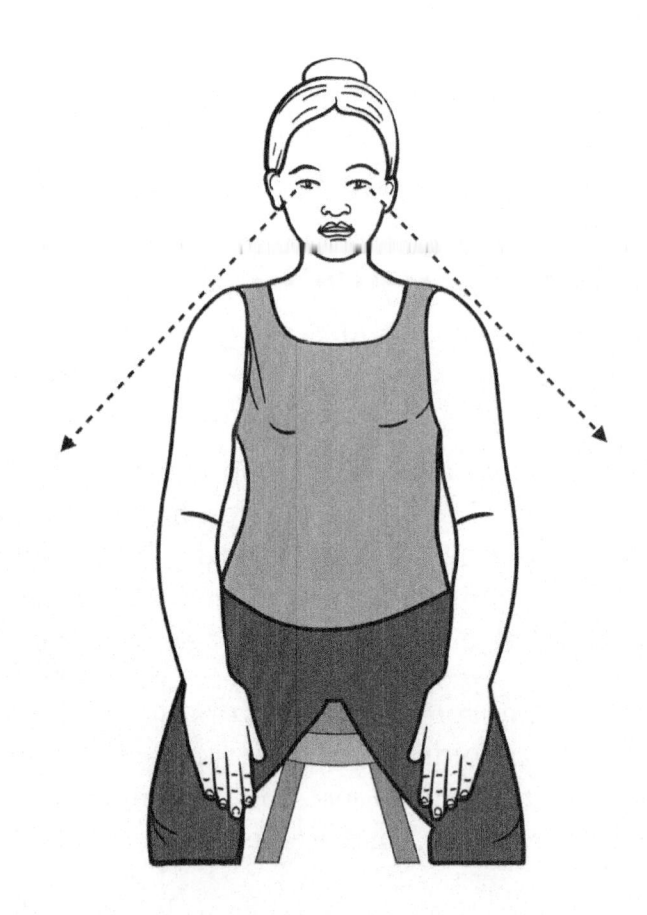

Level: Beginner

This simple exercise is a great way to release some of the tension in your eyes. Have you ever looked out at the horizon and allowed your eyes to take in the full view? This is known as "panoramic" vision, and it has incredible benefits. And it's not just about taking in pretty sights, either.

Believe it or not, how you view something can have an impact on your stress levels. If you are constantly zoned in, straining your eyes, you are adding to the stress on your body and mind. Finding ways to soften your gaze and open up your perception can have a significant impact.

For instance, should you see something that's exciting or stressful—for example, a stressful news headline—there is a real biological change happening. Your heart rate increases and your breathing becomes quicker and more shallow—but one of the most overlooked changes is in our vision itself! Our pupils automatically dilate, and the lens itself shifts, narrowing your field of vision (*How Panoramic Vision Can Reduce Your Stress and Anxiety*, 2022). Not only does this stress you out, but it causes significant eye strain. And you might not even realize that you're doing it.

According to neuroscientists, how we focus our eyes is linked to our internal stress levels. And our stress levels decrease when we're in panoramic vision. Panoramic vision opens the view, softening the gaze and allowing ourselves to focus on more at once. It mellows our fight-or-flight response and helps eye fatigue (*How Panoramic Vision Can Reduce Your Stress and Anxiety*, 2022). Give this a try the next time you are stressing out at your work computer.

1. **Keep looking straight ahead:** Or anywhere that feels comfortable.

2. **As you keep looking forward, open your gaze up and start to notice things in your periphery:** Notice what's going on at the edges of your peripheral vision. You don't want to focus on any one thing. Instead, allow yourself to notice it all. You want to give your eyes a rest here.

3. **As you do this, your gaze should soften.**

Workbook Exercises

1. As you opened up your vision wider, what did you notice?

2. When can you find moments throughout the day to practice this exercise?

Exercise 33: Cupping the Eyes

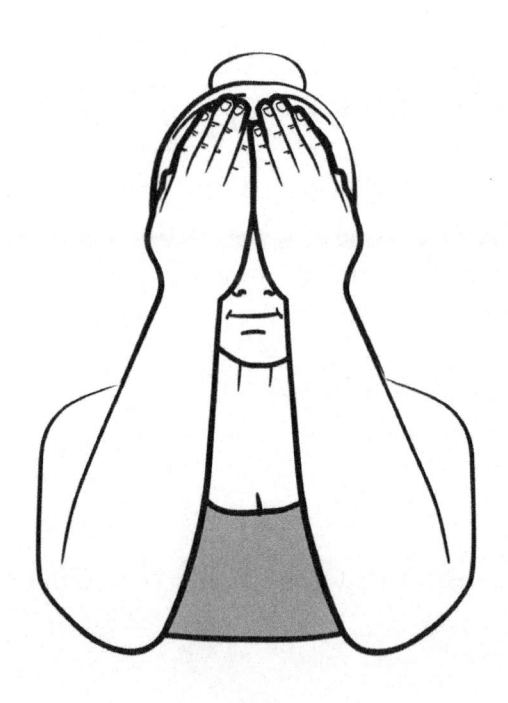

Level: Beginner

This exercise can be done standing, sitting, or lying down. It might seem simple, but this exercise can do wonders when it comes to relaxing your eyes and your entire nervous system. Though eye exercises are often forgotten, they have incredible benefits for your vision and lessen any potential eye strain. Doing exercises like these has been shown to prevent vision degeneration and even *improve* eyesight (Tomlinson, 2021). This exercise is effortless and relaxing, meaning it's not just helping your vision. It's also helping you find a moment of peace.

1. **Begin by rubbing your hands together vigorously:** This should generate heat between them.

2. **Cup your palms over your eyes gently:** Make sure you are *cupping* your hands over the eyes, not pressing your hands into the eyes.

3. **Take a few deep breaths:** Your eyes can either be open or closed for this.

4. **Allow the darkness to relax you:** Feel the tension leaving your body.

5. **After three to five minutes, gently let go:** Relax your arms as you do so.

Workbook Exercises

1. After doing this exercise, what sensations were you aware of?

2. Did you notice any changes in your vision?

Exercise 34: Release Neck and Shoulder Tension

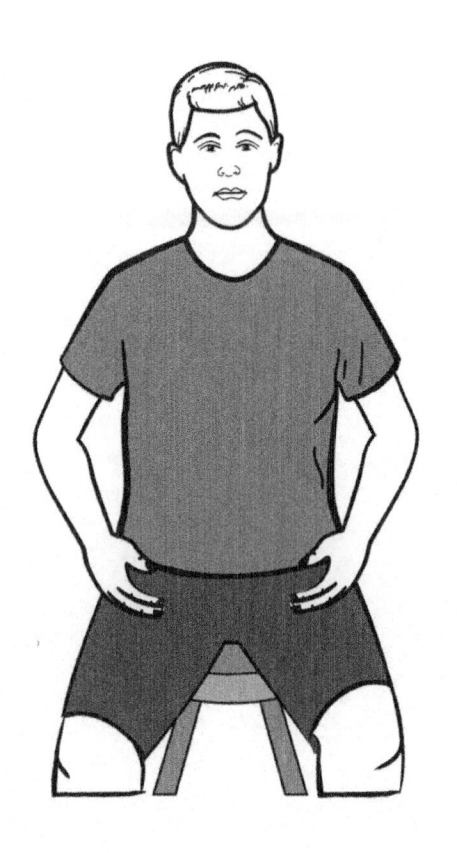

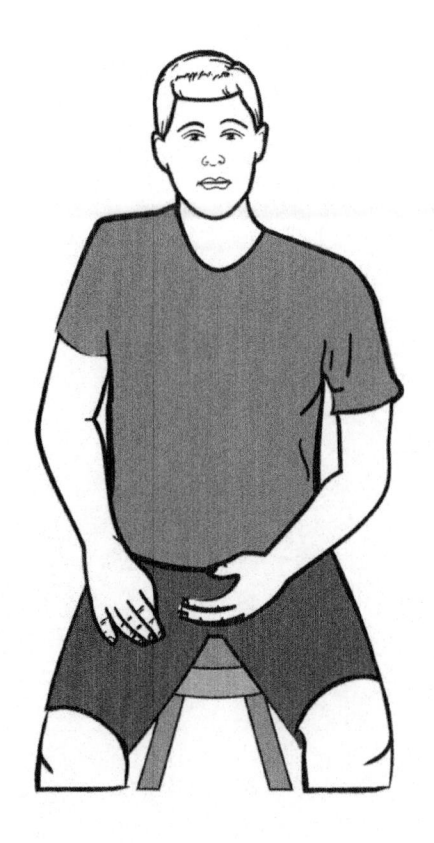

Level: Beginner

It's fairly common to hold tension in your neck and shoulders. This is often a chief complaint of those going to massage studios and chiropractors. There is a strong correlation between neck and shoulder pain and chronic stress (Ortego et al., 2016). When we begin to release the physical tension in our shoulders, it can actually impact our stress levels. This exercise is a simple way to do so.

This exercise isn't about the typical stretching or massaging you might have tried in the past. This is because stretching or massaging typically only helps for a short time. Eventually, the tension comes back. You keep having to stretch and massage constantly. This is because of the habitual use of your muscles—how you unconsciously move and hold yourself.

This exercise is about retraining and better understanding your nervous system. You aren't forcing your body to do something. Rather, you are helping your nervous system acknowledge the tension, making it easier to release.

1. **Start by checking your shoulder height:** Which shoulder is higher than the other? What is the distance between the ears and the shoulders?

2. **Slowly raise your right shoulder:** Take about 10 seconds to get there.

3. **Once you get there, stay there for 10 seconds:** Feel the effort it takes to hold it there.

4. **Now, very slowly bring your shoulder back down:** Release that effort and strain as you do so.

5. **Check the height of the shoulders again:** Is anything different?

6. **Repeat on the other shoulder.**

Workbook Exercises

1. Before the exercises, how did your neck and shoulders feel?

2. Take inventory of how stressed you feel at the moment.

3. After the exercise, how did you feel emotionally? What sensations did you feel in your body?

Exercise 35: Retraining the Neck and Shoulders

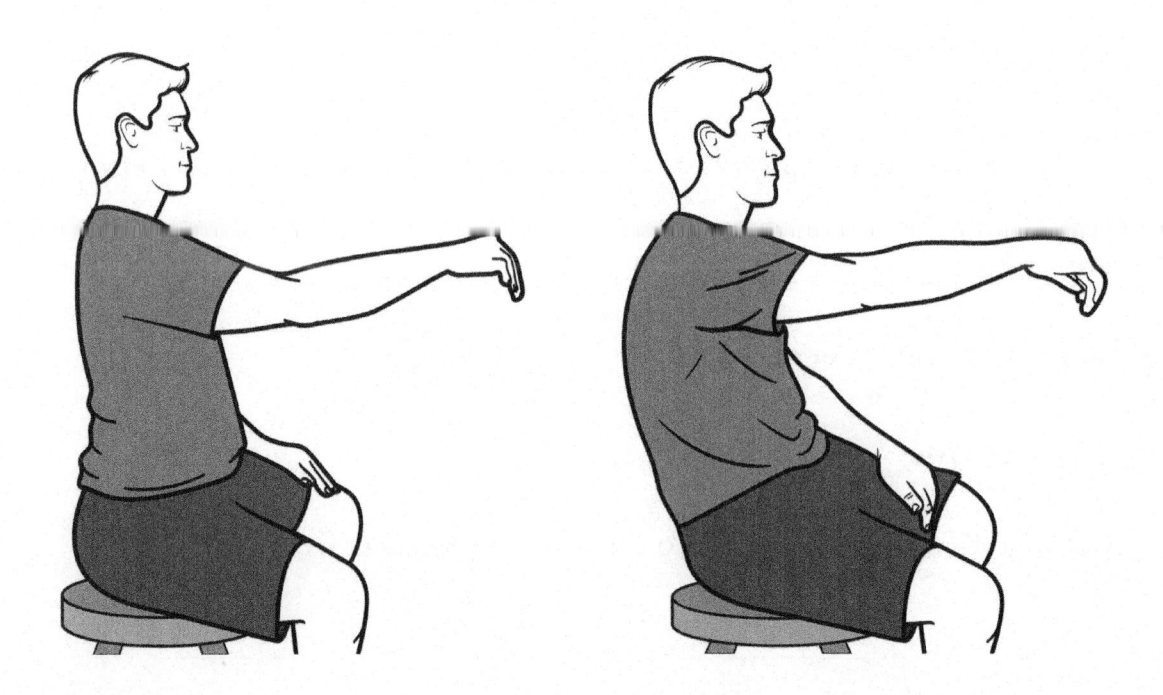

Level: Intermediate

This awareness exercise can make a world of difference in the tension you hold in your neck and shoulders. Incorporating this practice might mean saying goodbye to chronic muscle strain and tension in that area. And it only takes a few moments out of your day.

Remember, this is how we are retraining our nervous system. We are bringing awareness to our habitual muscle use. When we acknowledge it, we are allowing our nervous system the chance to make changes.

Stress can often mean pain in certain areas of our body. It makes sense, as a tense mind will often mean a tense body. That mind–body connection works in both positive and negative ways. But we can retrain our neck and shoulders to release some of that tension and, in doing so, release some of that stress.

1. **Sit in a chair with a comfortable but neutral stance.**

2. **Bring one arm up to about shoulder height:** Ensure that your arms are loose by your sides.

3. **From that position, roll your pelvis backward:** You want to round your back as you do so.

4. **Notice the distance between the shoulder and the ear:** The shoulder will have come up closer to the ear.

5. **Roll the pelvis slightly forward, lengthening the spine.**

6. **Again, notice the distance between the shoulder and the ear:** It will have increased with this shift in posture.

7. **Repeat this series of movements three to five times for each arm.**

Note: *Pay attention to your body and go through these motions slowly.*

Workbook Exercises

1. After the exercise, without trying to analyze what happened, how has your mental and emotional state shifted?

2. How might you incorporate this exercise into your daily routine?

Exercise 36: Progressive Muscle Relaxation

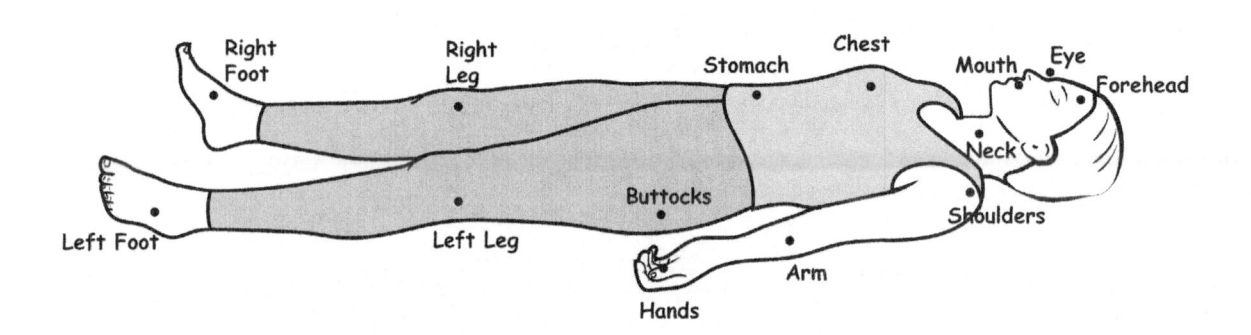

Level: Beginner

Progressive muscle relaxation is a simple way to bring your attention to the areas in your body where there is tension, and to systematically release that tension. Modern research has found that this exercise not only positively impacts your mental health but also provides better quality sleep and lowers blood pressure (Toussaint et al., 2021).

This exercise is best done lying down, but you can try it sitting as well. I know several people who incorporate this into their routine by practicing it right before bed. The release of tension is a great way to set yourself up for a good night's rest.

1. **Begin by finding a comfortable position:** It's usually best if you can lie down.

2. **Close or half close your eyes.**

3. **Focus on how you are breathing out, and relax.**

4. **Focus on your feet:** Curl your toes under and tense your feet as hard as you can for five counts, before releasing the tension.

5. **Notice how the muscles there are feeling looser.**

6. **Tense the muscles in your legs as hard as you can:** Tense those muscles for five counts, before releasing the tension.

7. **Feel how much looser and less tense those muscles are now.**

8. **Tense the muscles in your arms and hands:** Clench your fists and flex your biceps for a count of five, before releasing that tension.

9. **Bring your shoulders to your ears and tense your shoulder muscles:** Count five counts and release that tension.

10. **Feel the muscles in your neck and shoulders relax.**

11. **Tense your facial muscles:** Hold for five counts before releasing the tension.

12. **Feel all the muscles in your face relax.**

13. **Start to wiggle your fingers and toes:** As you do so, open your eyes and end the exercise.

Workbook Exercises

1. In which muscle group did you notice the most tension?

2. How did you feel in your body after the exercise?

Exercise 37: Release Psoas

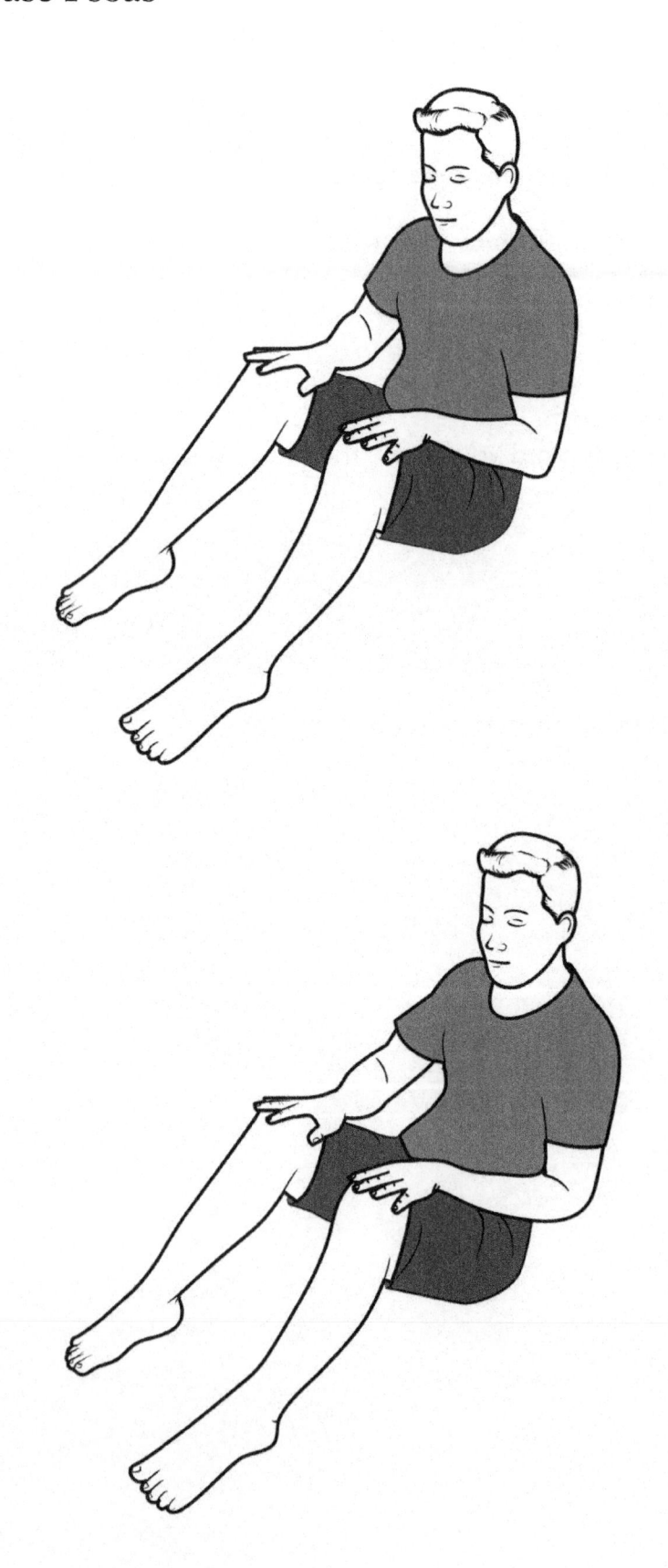

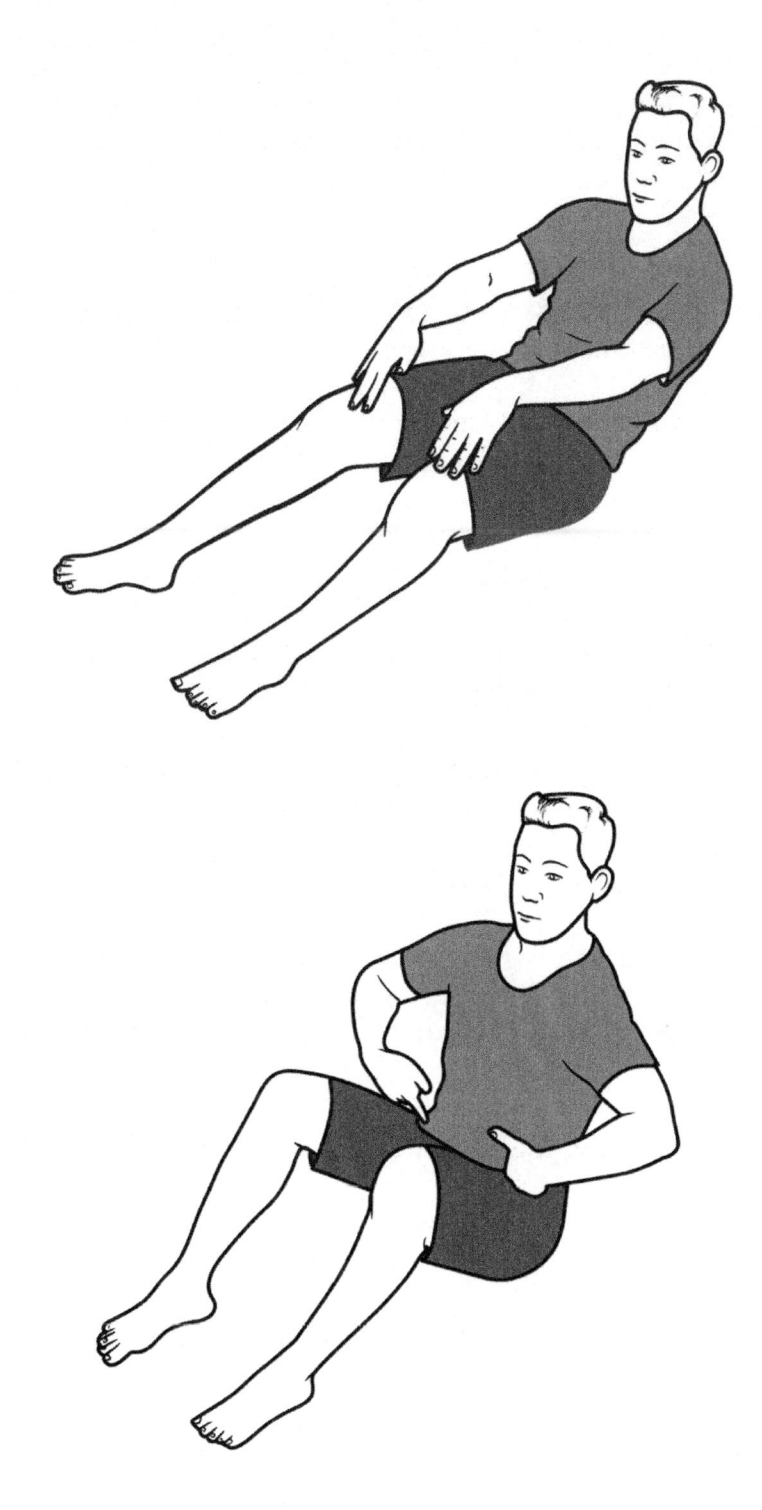

Level: Intermediate

Hip flexibility might not seem that important, but researchers have discovered that it has a much greater impact beyond physical fitness. When we are discussing releasing tension in the body, there's likely no muscle group more important in the management of PTSD than the psoas major. This muscle group in the hip region is one of the principal contributors to psychosomatic experiences and the reactive stress system. It is likely involved in both the development and relief of PTSD (Siccardi et al., 2020).

This exercise will help you relax tension and encourage flexibility in the psoas major muscle group, while also encouraging you along your somatic healing journey. This is a more intermediate exercise, and special care should be taken if you have any injuries or health considerations.

1. **Lie flat on the floor with your legs out straight and your arms lying by your sides:** Notice the space behind your back. Take note of the curvature in your spine—the space between the spine and the ground.

2. **Now, sit up:** You want your feet flat on the ground in front of you. If you have a hard time with this, put a cushion underneath your glutes or pelvis for added support. Make sure your pelvis is rolled forward. You want to be upright.

3. **Place your palms on your thighs:** Let them rest just above the knees.

4. **Now, slowly roll your pelvis backward and start leaning back:** You want your spine to round somewhat.

5. **As you do so, slide your feet away from you:** You will be lengthening your legs and engaging your abdominal muscles.

6. **Using your hip flexor muscles, start sliding your feet back toward you.**

7. **As you do so, pull your pelvis forward:** This should lengthen your spine.

8. **Stay in this position for five seconds:** You should be feeling an engagement of the hip flexor muscles.

9. **Slowly let go, sliding your feet away from you and rolling your pelvis back:** You should be rounding your spine.

10. **Repeat three more times.**

11. **Slowly lie down, and recheck that space behind your back:** Has it lessened?

Workbook Exercises

1. On a scale from 1 to 10, how tight were your psoas muscles before the exercise? After?

2. Try walking around the room. How different does it feel to walk with the psoas relaxed?

Exercise 38: Release Stomach Tension

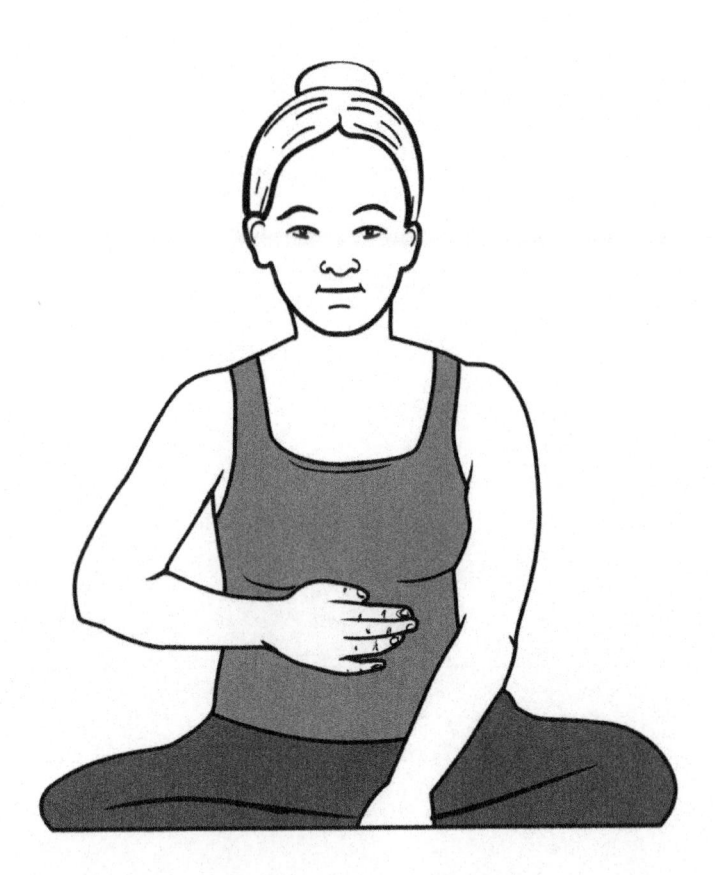

Level: Beginner

This exercise is about letting go—not just of tension but of emotions. Have you ever wanted to let something go, but you just couldn't? Perhaps it was anger over an argument or frustration over a lost opportunity. Despite your resolution, you found yourself hanging on to that emotion long after the event. It weighed you down and robbed you of your joy and focus on anything else.

Likewise, you might feel tension in your body without truly understanding what the emotion is. This scenario can be particularly frustrating because it can be difficult to address an emotion you can't identify. Of course, as we've learned, there *are* exercises for dealing with emotions we don't quite understand. They allow us to center ourselves, activate the parasympathetic nervous system, and resolve any frustrating emotions that linger. We often do this by activating the vagus nerve.

The vagus nerve extends down into the abdomen, so by releasing the tension there, you are allowing it to better activate. Activating the vagus nerve triggers a calmer, more regulated state. In this exercise, we activate it by pumping the diaphragm and relaxing the stomach as a whole. This should make you feel a sense of release, as well as more relaxed in both body and mind.

1. **Find a comfortable seated position:** Make sure your spine is lengthened and straight. If you are seated in a chair, make sure your feet are flat on the floor.

2. **Close your eyes and take a deep inhale through your nose.**

3. **Hold your breath for a few counts.**

4. **As you do so, pump your diaphragm:** Do this by pulling in your upper abdominal muscles, then relaxing them over and over again.

5. **Continue pumping your diaphragm until you need to exhale.**

6. **Exhale through your nose.**

7. **Repeat:** You can repeat for three to five minutes, or for as long as you are comfortable. It might be helpful to put your right hand on your diaphragm area to feel the motion of your diaphragm pumping.

Workbook Exercises

1. Did you have challenges relaxing the belly? Describe why it might be challenging for you.

2. What happened when you finally allowed yourself to release your stomach?

Exercise 39: Psoas Pandiculation

Level: Intermediate

Have you ever woken up from a good sleep, stretching and yawning as you did so? This is the act of pandiculation. That stretch and yawn is a fundamental part of your neuromuscular functioning (Toner, n.d.). It is how our nervous system naturally wakes up our sensorimotor system and prepares us for movement. While this motion might *look* like a stretch, it's actually us contracting muscles that have stayed inactive for a while (Warren, 2022).

Pandiculation is a term coined by Thomas Hanna, and it refers to re-educating the neuromuscular system. It is also the best way to release any tightness in the psoas muscle. This is done through active movement.

Because the psoas muscle group is so large and central, when it is tight, it can lead to a number of painful conditions. This can look like pain or spasms in the lower back, lumbar disc problems, idiopathic scoliosis, sciatica, and more. With all these potential downfalls of a tight psoas region, it's important to focus on loosening these muscles. This exercise helps you do this through pandiculation, which already comes naturally to the body.

Exercise 1

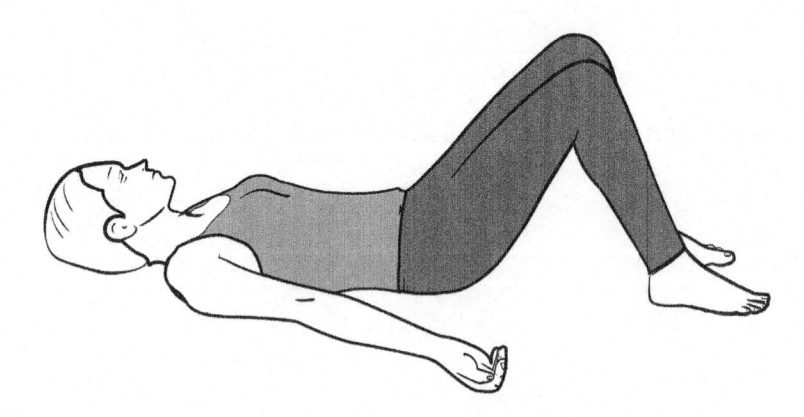

1. **Start by standing up:** Stand normally, letting your arms hang by your sides. Don't try to have perfect posture.

2. **Close your eyes:** Take a few moments to breathe, and notice how your body feels today.

3. **Bring your awareness to your lower back:** Are there any areas of pain or tightness? Is your pelvis straight up and down, or more out or under? Just notice. Don't try to change anything.

4. **Come down to the floor, lying down on your back:** Bend your knees, keeping your feet and knees a comfortable hip-width apart.

5. **Close your eyes again and notice how your lower back feels in this position.**

6. **Start bringing your attention to your breath:** Begin taking deep breaths into your lower belly. Perhaps put your hands over your lower abdomen to feel your diaphragm expanding and contracting.

7. **Slowly press the base of your spine down toward the floor three times:** This is to get you used to moving this area.

8. **When you're ready, inhale into your belly and press the base of your spine down into the floor.**

9. **Keep pressing gently, and slowly start rolling that pressure toward your belly.**

10. **Slowly start exhaling and releasing that pressure, letting it roll back to neutral:** This should feel like a release of tension, allowing you to float back down to the floor.

11. **Rest before doing the movement again.**

12. **Repeat.**

Exercise 2

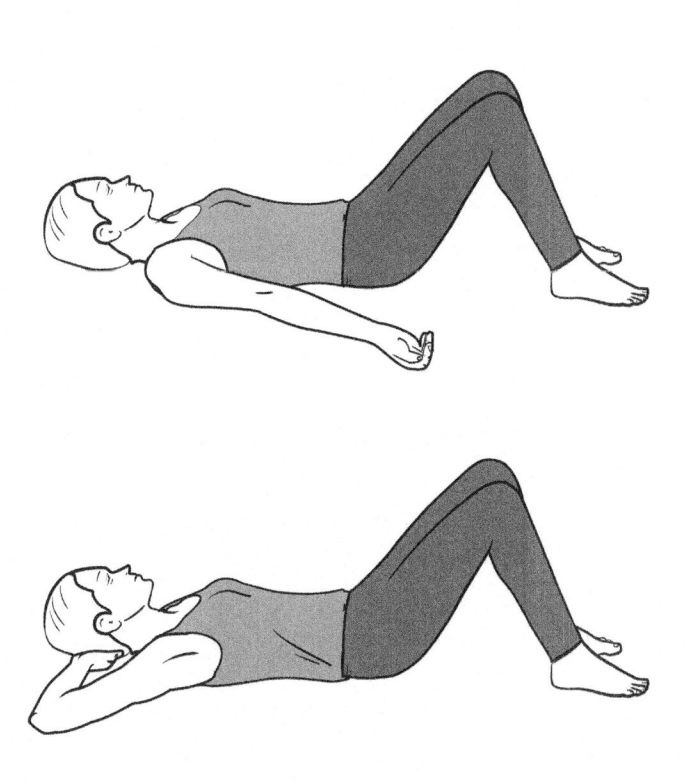

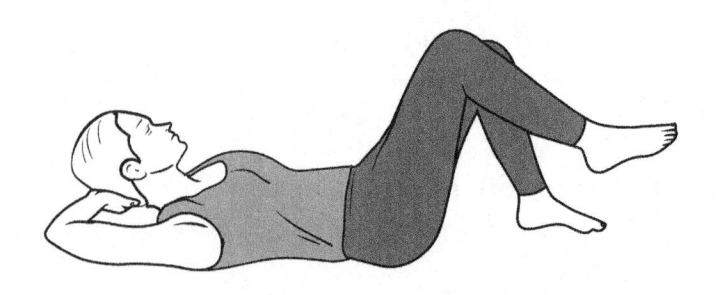

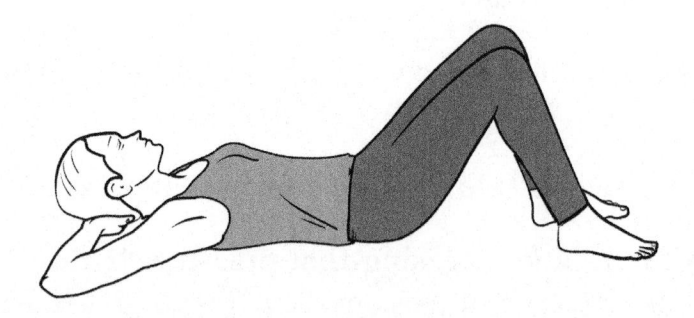

1. **Bring yourself back to a neutral, lying-down position, knees bent, feet flat on the ground, and take a few deep breaths:** You want to rest before tackling this next exercise.

2. **Keep your lower back flattened to the ground throughout the entire exercise:** This will engage the iliopsoas.

3. **Rest your head in the palm of your right hand, letting your right elbow bend out to the side:** You can allow your left arm to rest at your side.

4. **Take a big inhale down into your belly.**

5. **As you slowly exhale, press your lower back firmly into the floor.**

6. **Now, lift up your head so you are curling up:** At the same time, lift up your right leg. Keep the knees bent.

7. **Keep lowering your lower back down into the floor, and lower your head and leg back down:** Do this at a slow pace. You want to have as much control as you can. Be careful not to strain or overuse your neck muscles. Allow your right hand to gently support the weight of your head.

8. **Be careful not to strain or overuse your neck muscles:** Allow your right hand to gently support your neck.

9. **When your foot hits the floor, release your lower back and take a moment to relax.**

10. **Repeat these steps on the left side.**

Workbook Exercises

1. On a scale of 1–10, how much pain did you have before the exercise? After?

2. Try walking around the room. How different does it feel to walk with the psoas released?

Activating the Vagus Nerve

You might have noticed a quick mention of "the vagus nerve" in a previous exercise. The vagus nerve is basically an information superhighway to our brain. It sends and receives information to help regulate the parasympathetic nervous system and all the operations that it controls—from digestion and heart rate to mood and the body's inflammation system (Paturel, 2024).

However, just like our muscles, we need to keep our nerves active for them to work optimally. This includes the vagus nerve. The exercises to activate this nerve and keep it healthy aren't like the workouts you might get at a gym, but their benefits to your health are comparable. When you regularly activate and care for the vagus nerve, you might experience benefits such as better mood, better sleep, lowered blood pressure and heart rate, and even less pain and inflammation in the body (Mayo Clinic Staff, 2023).

Toning the vagus nerve is a lot like toning any muscle group. You want to activate and use it. This can look different from exercise to exercise. You might find yourself accessing it through movement or through directly stimulating the nerve.

Throughout these exercises, we will focus on this important nerve. While some of these exercises might feel simple, they are actually having a profound impact on your parasympathetic nervous system and multiple bodily functions.

Exercise 40: Ear Pull

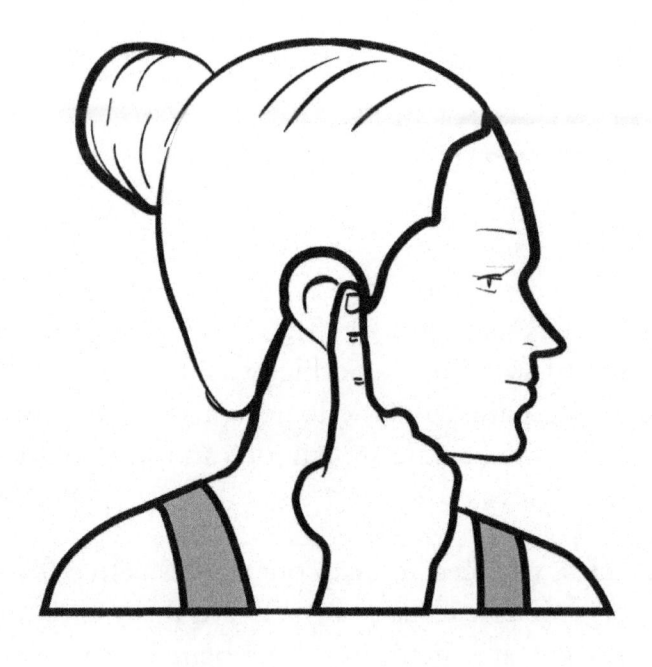

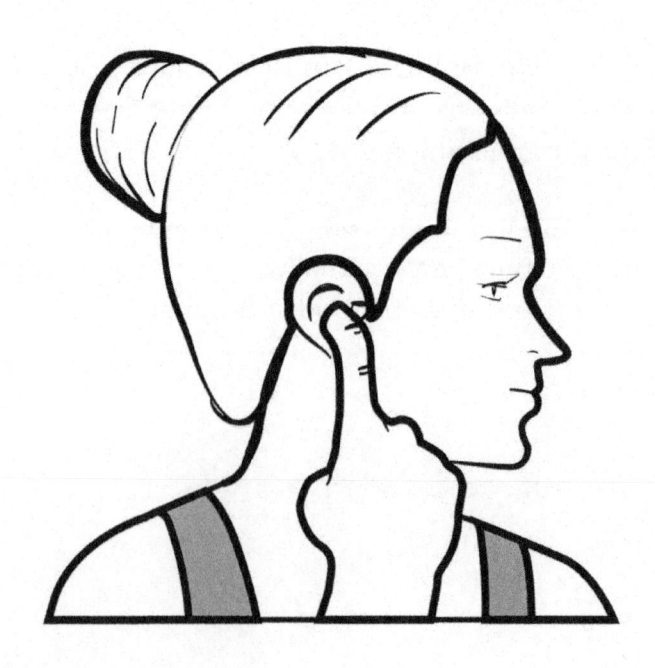

Level: Beginner

This exercise regulates your nervous system by activating the vagus nerve. From the outside, it might look simple, but it can greatly impact any feelings of anxiety or dysregulation.

Anxiety has an intense response inside the body. From muscle tension to digestion issues, you can *feel* the chain of events happening in your body. To ease those anxious feelings, try this exercise to calm the nervous system and bring yourself back to center.

1. **Place your left finger inside your left ear:** Put it toward the bottom, inserting it gently.

2. **Gently pull down the ear:** When you pull down like this, you are actually activating the vagus nerve.

3. **Breathe slowly and deeply for about 20 seconds:** Focus in on your breaths, inhaling through the nose and exhaling through the mouth.

4. **Pause and check in with yourself:** How do you feel?

5. **Repeat steps 1–3 with the opposite ear and finger.**

Workbook Exercises

1. Did you notice any sensations in your body while doing the exercise?

2. Where can you integrate this exercise into your everyday life (e.g., during breaks, before sleeping, after you park the car)?

Exercise 41: Salamander Exercise

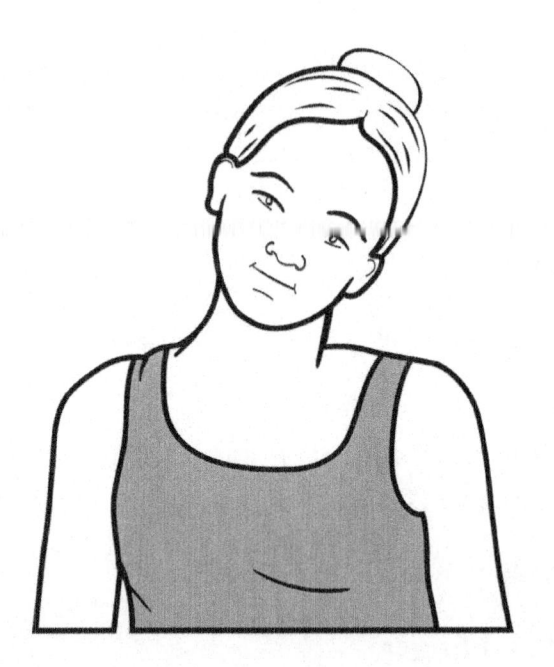

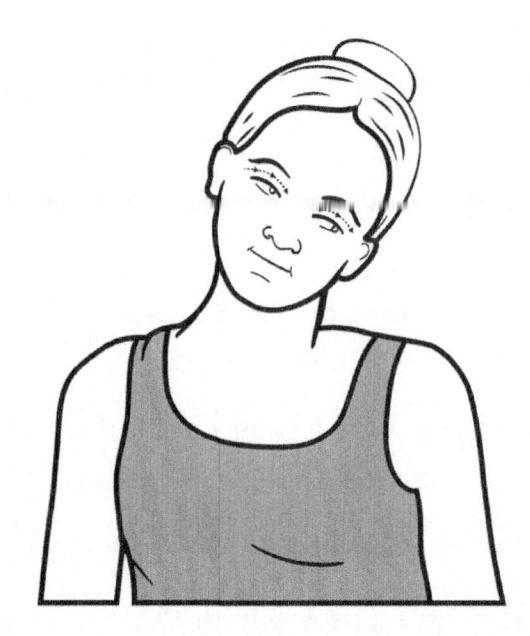

Level: Beginner

When you have experienced trauma, it can be easy to get locked in a state of fight or flight. Everything seems like a threat, and you are in constant protection mode. However, when we are so focused on protection, we can't fully focus on our healing and growth. It becomes imperative, then, to step out of that constant threat mode and into a more balanced approach.

This exercise is called the Salamander Exercise because it helps us move away from the "reptilian brain" that keeps us stuck in fight or flight. It allows us to step into a place of more gentle calm and healing, if only for a moment. As you continue to practice this technique, you will find it easier to step out of those moments and re-center yourself.

As you participate in this technique, ensure that you are listening to your body and going slowly. This exercise can cause the release of emotions, and you don't want to overwhelm yourself.

1. **Tilt your head to the side:** The ear should go straight toward the shoulder. Don't look down. Keep your eyes forward. Depending on your range of motion, your head might only move a few degrees. That's okay! Keep your head tilted for 30 seconds on each side.

2. **Now, look straight to the left with just your eyes:** Now that you are back to center, just look to your three o'clock, straight to the left.

3. **Combine the side-to-side motion with the eye movement:** Look straight to the left as you tilt your head as you did in step 1.

4. **Repeat steps 2 and 3, now looking to the right.**

5. **Keep going until you sense a kind of release:** This might be a yawn, a swallow, or even an emotional release.

Workbook Exercises

1. How did your body respond to this exercise (e.g., yawning, swallowing, emotional release)?

2. Notice the level of tension in your body before and after the exercise. Do you notice any difference?

Exercise 42: Vagus Nerve Activation Routine

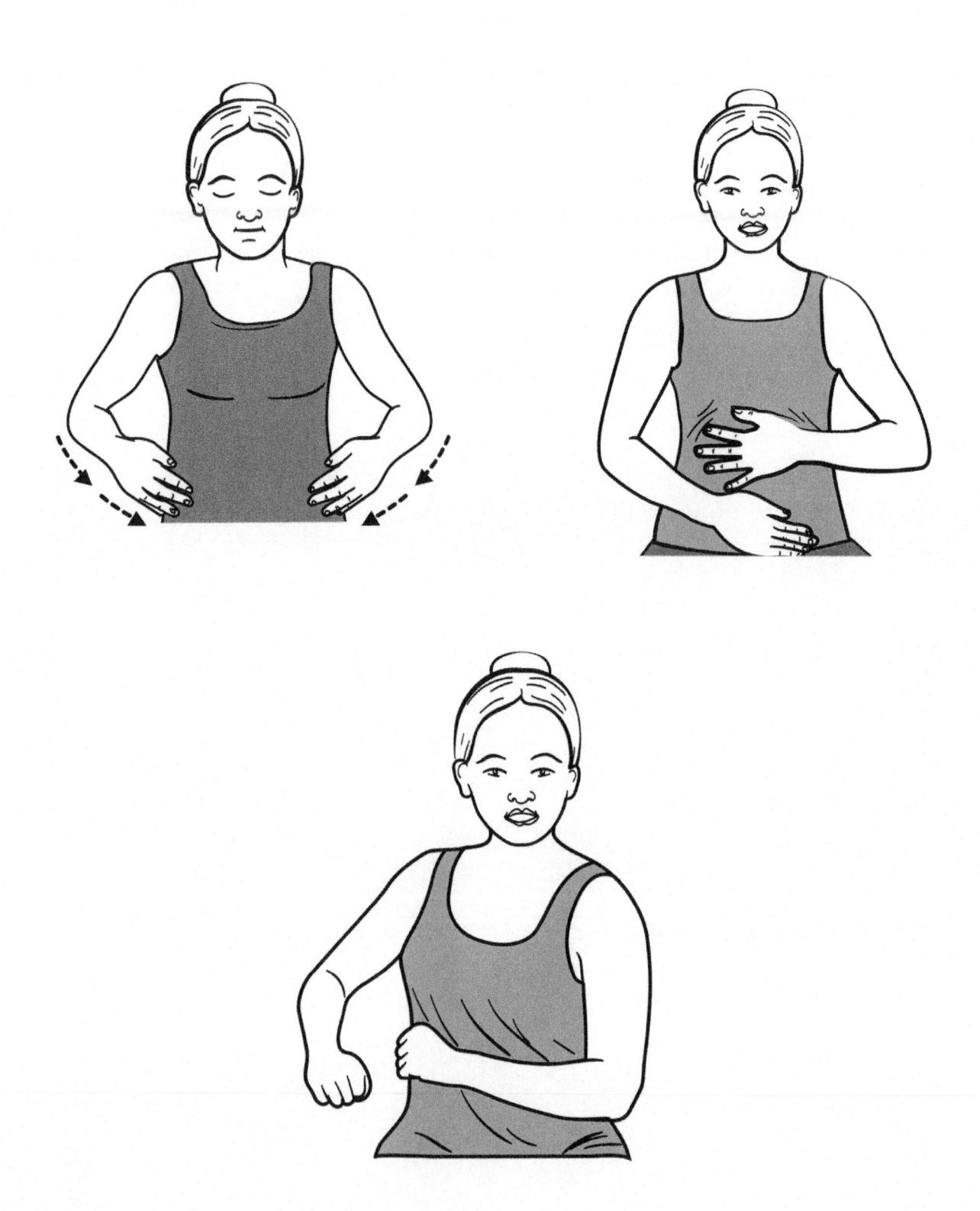

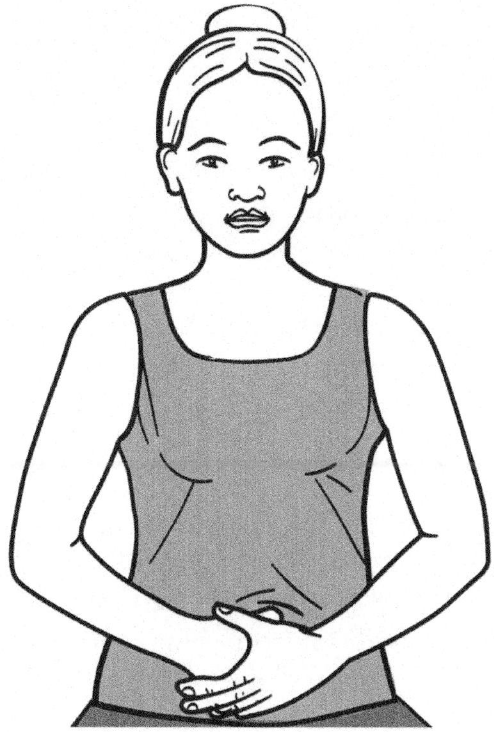

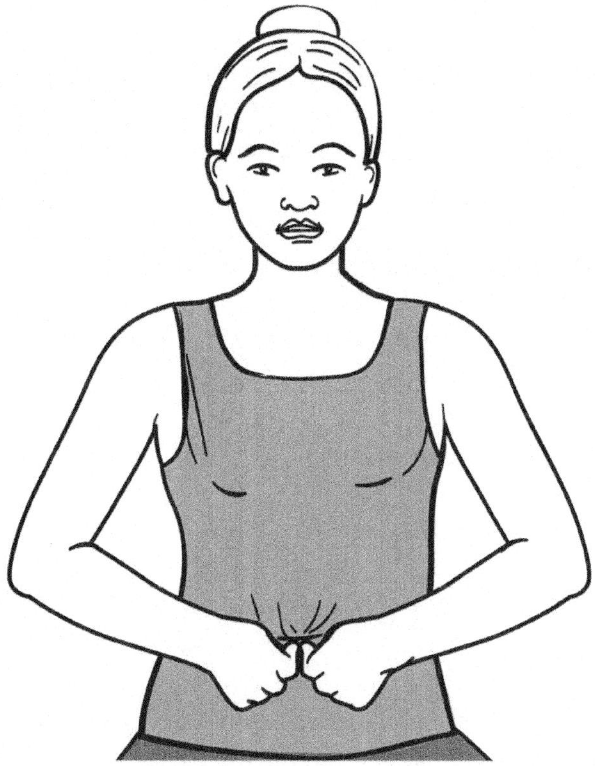

Level: Beginner

Many of our activities engage the vagus nerve in some way. That is because our vagus nerve is connected to so many bodily processes. It checks in on our organs to ensure that everything is running properly and smoothly. And, of course, it helps us relax by activating the parasympathetic nervous system. Probably one of the best ways to activate this nerve is through this next exercise.

What I love about this exercise is its accessibility. It surprises a lot of people to learn that we can get so much benefit out of an exercise that isn't super rigorous. Instead, we are tuning into our body and engaging our system gently.

1. **Start by taking a seat:** Have your feet flat on the ground, keeping your spine straight. Tuck your chin slightly inward, and relax your shoulders.

2. **Tap your abdomen 30 times with both hands:** You should be tapping the lower belly, right underneath your belly button. This will open up that area to stimulate the vagus nerve.

3. **Now, place your right hand on your belly button and your left hand right above it:** Tap both areas simultaneously 50 times. You might feel some pain in your solar plexus. If you do, exhale. Relax your gut.

4. **Rub your belly in circles with both hands:** It should feel like a light massage.

5. **Put your hands in front of you with your elbows bent, fists facing each other, and twist side to side:** You are opening your midsection. Do this 30 times.

6. Now that you are all opened up, it's time to stimulate the vagus nerve.

7. **Stack your hands on top of each other, dominant hand underneath:** The dominant hand should stick up its thumb and push it into your belly button.

8. **Do little pumps into your belly button:** Do this 30 times.

9. **Now, pump into your belly button with *both* thumbs:** Do this 30 times.

10. **Pump into your belly button with the pointer and middle fingers of both hands:** Do this 30 times.

11. **Rest your hands on your knees and close your eyes:** Feel the changes in your body as opposed to before. Do you feel warmer? Do you feel tingly? Do you feel saliva in your mouth? Maybe a slight sense of calmness and centeredness in your brain?

12. **Take a few deep breaths:** Inhale through your nose and exhale through your mouth. What changes do you feel? Any lessening of tension in the gut?

Workbook Exercises

1. What kind of emotional response did you have from this exercise?

2. After the emotions settled, how did you feel?

Exercise 43: Polyvagal Vagus Nerve Reset

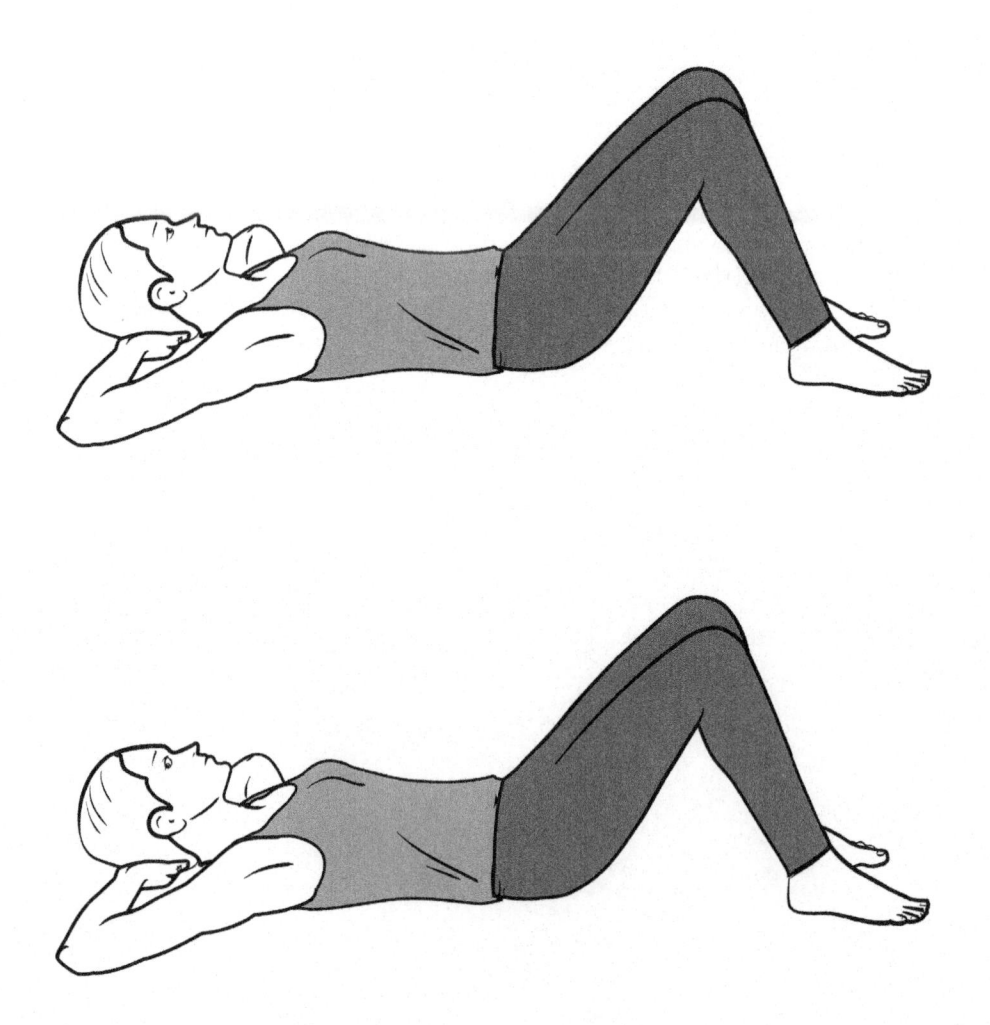

Level: Beginner

Like the last exercise, this one doesn't require much movement. This activity can be quite activating. Make sure that you are taking care of yourself as you venture into this practice. Ease into it, and listen to your body. There's no rush.

This exercise operates based on polyvagal theory. This theory encompasses how the vagus nerve, the autonomic nervous system, and the central nervous system come together to regulate several responses, from the fear response to emotional regulation. When we consider this connection, we can use it to our advantage, healing the trauma we experience.

Trauma is not necessarily about what happened to you. It's how your nervous system was rewired in the wake of the events. That is why we're spending so much time discussing the reworking of the nervous system. It's the fastest and most effective way to relieve feelings of anxiety and stress, especially those brought on by trauma.

In this next exercise, I will help you reset the vagus nerve, relieving not just anxiety and stress but pain and tension as well. (Remember, they are inextricably linked!) Again, ensure that you are easing into the practice, as this can stir up some emotional responses.

1. **Get in a comfortable position:** Sit up with your back lengthened and straight.

2. **Turn your head side to side:** Notice if it's easier to turn in one direction or the other. This gives us our baseline.

3. **Lie down:** It is best to practice this technique lying down at first, though once you have mastered it, you can do it sitting up. Bend your knees, feet flat on the floor.

4. **Interlace your fingers and place your hands behind your head:** You'll be cradling your head.

5. **Move your eyes to the right while keeping your head straight:** Your nose should remain pointing up as you look to the right. Stay there for 30 seconds.

6. **Bring your eyes back to the middle:** Notice what is happening in your body.

7. **Now, move your eyes to the left, head still pointing straight:** Stay there for another 30 seconds.

8. **After the activity, sit up and test your mobility again:** What has changed in your body and your mobility since the beginning of the exercise?

Workbook Exercises

1. What kind of emotional response did you have to this activity?

2. After the emotions settled, how did you feel?

Exercise 44: Butterfly Hug

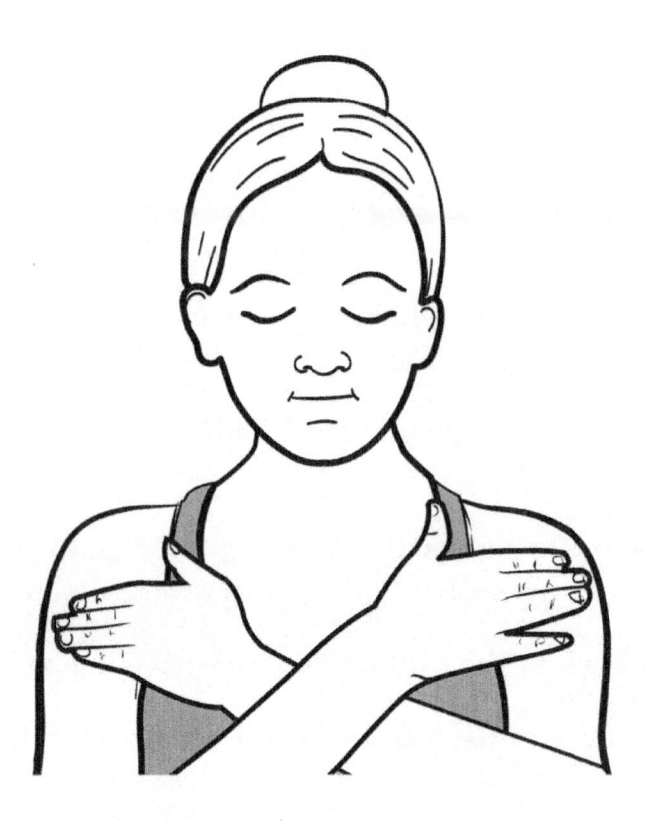

Level: Beginner

Earlier, we discussed bilateral stimulation and its impact on the brain. You might be surprised to find that it has a significant impact on the vagus nerve as well. This special type of bilateral stimulation soothes our nervous system and brings us back to center. If you ever find yourself in a situation where you need to calm down or re-regulate your system, this is a great exercise to practice.

With this activity, you can soothe and release some of the tension in your body. This will then send a signal to your brain that you are safe. It will not only calm those trauma and anxiety symptoms; it will also start retraining your brain in how it reacts to whatever stimuli set you off in the first place (Filipiak, n.d.).

1. **First, find a safe, quiet place:** This might be a favorite chair or a quiet hallway—anywhere that is away from others and allows you some peace and quiet.

2. **Sit up straight:** You want your spine to be lengthened and straight, your head lightly resting above it.

3. **Close your eyes if you are comfortable:** If you aren't comfortable with this, just lower your gaze.

4. **Take some deep, purposeful breaths:** If possible, try breathing from your diaphragm.

5. **Notice any distress that might be coming up:** And try to just breathe through it, as far as you can.

6. **Cross your hands across your chest, with each middle finger lying just beneath the opposite collarbone:** Fan out your fingers, with your thumb pointing toward your chin.

7. **Now, interlock your thumbs:** See how your hands now look like a butterfly?

8. **Now, take turns tapping on your chest:** Do this one hand at a time, slowly and rhythmically. You should go for about eight rounds. Breathe purposefully as you do so.

9. **Stop and check in on your distress:** If you aren't feeling any more distressed, try going for another round of eight. After each set, stop and check your distress.

Workbook Exercises

1. What kind of emotional response did you have to this exercise?

2. After the emotions settled, how did you feel?

Exercise 45: Hand Reflexology

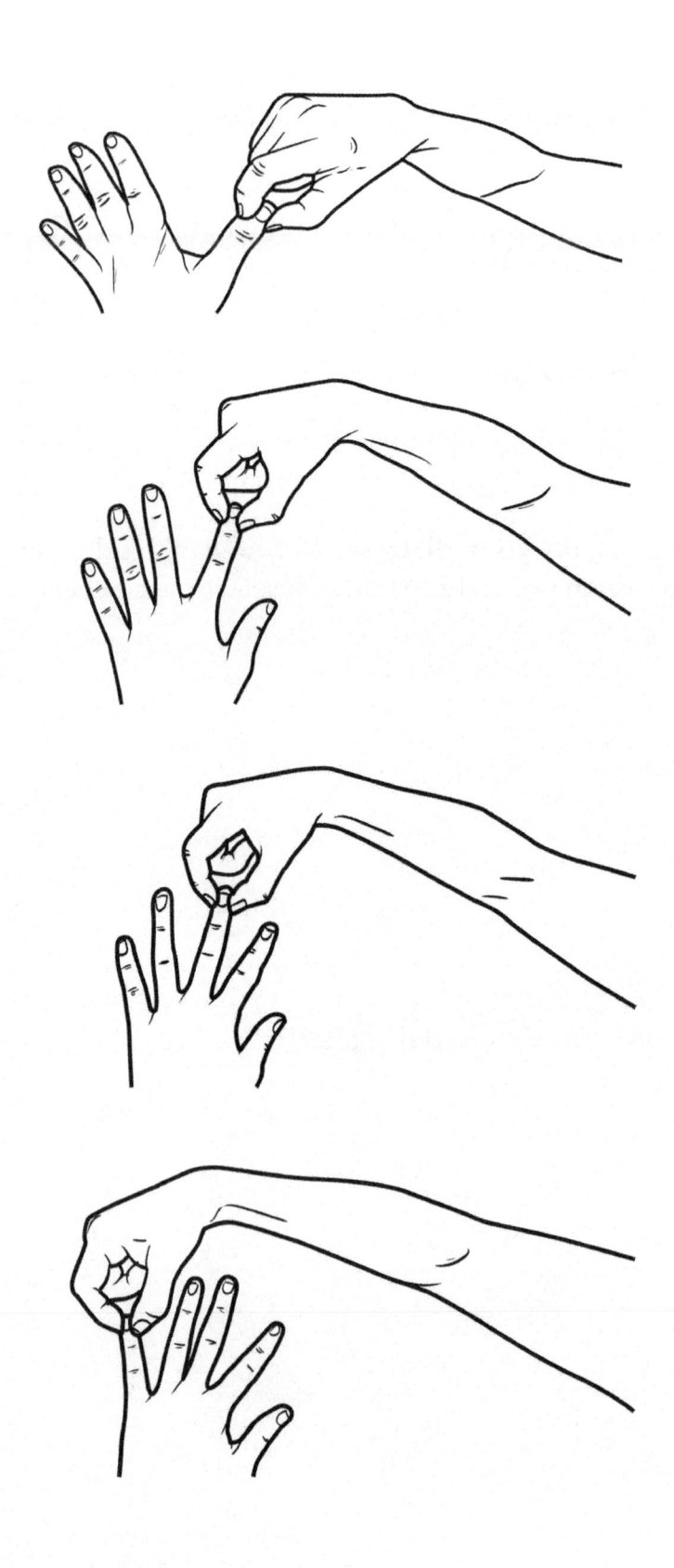

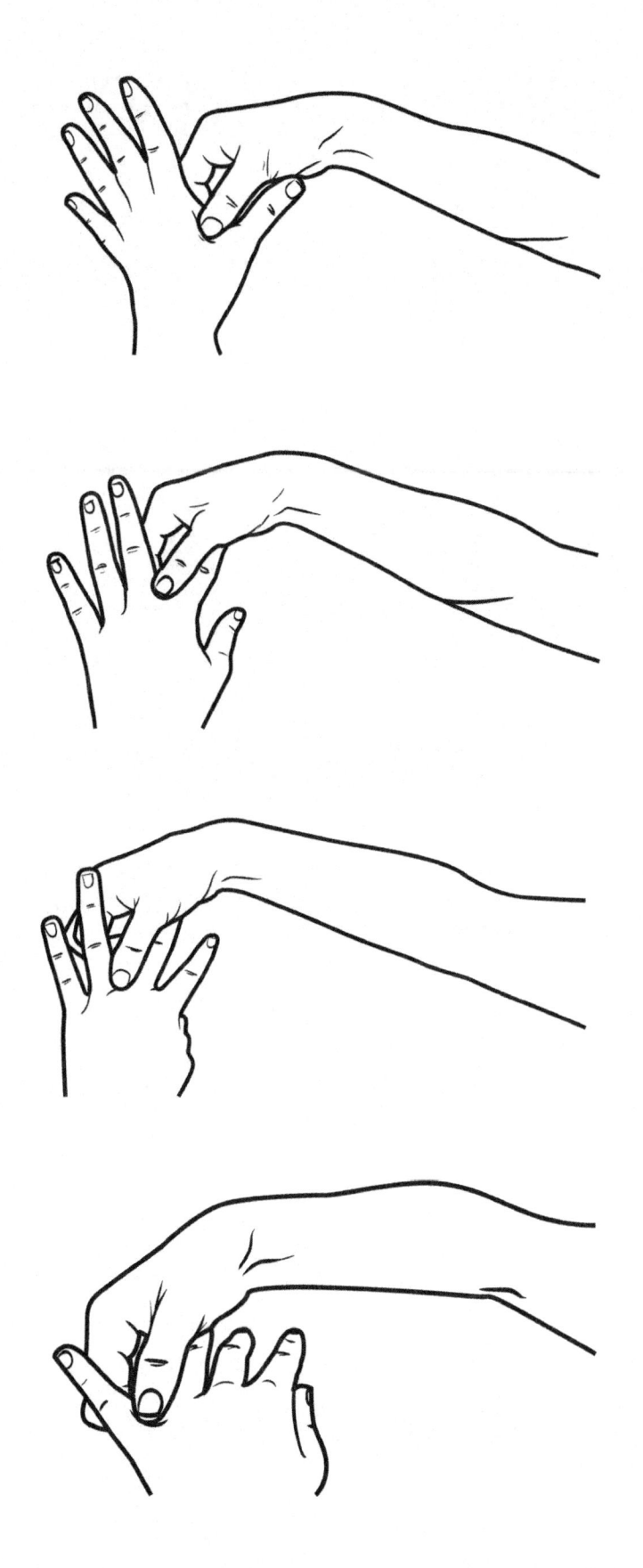

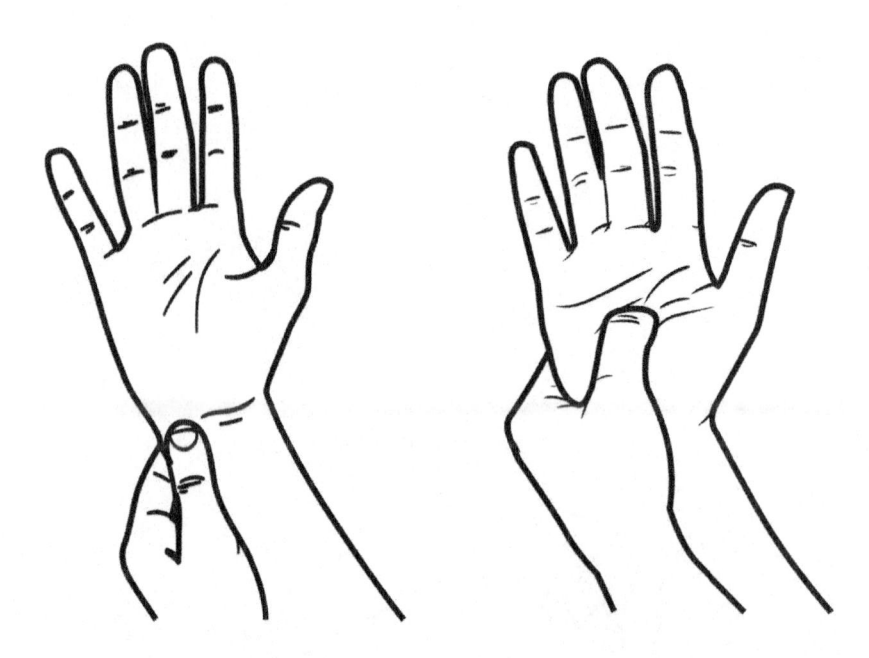

Level: Beginner

Hand reflexology doesn't take a lot of movement, so it might seem to the untrained eye like nothing is happening. However, research has shown that this seemingly simple technique can actually improve pain and fatigue (Cronkleton, 2018). Much of that effect is owed to the mind–body connection. We are stimulating the vagus nerve when we practice this technique, bringing out the parasympathetic nervous system. When it sends out those relaxing signals, we find ourselves easing out of anxiety and pain.

Studies have found some amazing applications for hand reflexology. For instance, researchers have discovered that this practice can ease pain and fatigue following a coronary angiography (Ortego et al., 2016). This suggests further, more extensive applications when it comes to fatigue and pain in patients.

1. **Pinch each side of the nail bed—the skin beneath the nail plate—10 times:** Or squeeze for 10 seconds each. This will stimulate the pressure points there.

2. **Repeat on all fingers, except the ring finger:** This is because the ring finger activates the sympathetic nervous system. Only use the ring finger if you feel that you are down or depressed, or if you have low blood sugar or low blood pressure. Otherwise, you want to encourage relaxation by skipping that finger.

3. **Repeat on the other hand.**

4. **Massage the webbing between each finger and then pinch each time before moving onto the next one:** After pinching, slide out, keeping your fingers pinched.

5. **Now, draw a line from the base of your ring and pinky finger down to your wrist:** Where it stops on the wrist crease is another pressure point. (This is called heart 7 or H7.)

6. **Press that point for five seconds as you take deep breaths:** Repeat this five times. This helps with emotional distress, insomnia, overthinking, and anxiety.

7. **Now, make a thumbs-up:** The next pressure point is where your middle finger is touching your palm.

8. **Press this point for five seconds as you take deep breaths.**

9. **Repeat five times.**

Workbook Exercises

1. On a scale of 1–10, what was your anxiety level before the exercise? After?

2. Bring attention to your breathing. How has it changed after the exercise?

Exercise 46: Humming

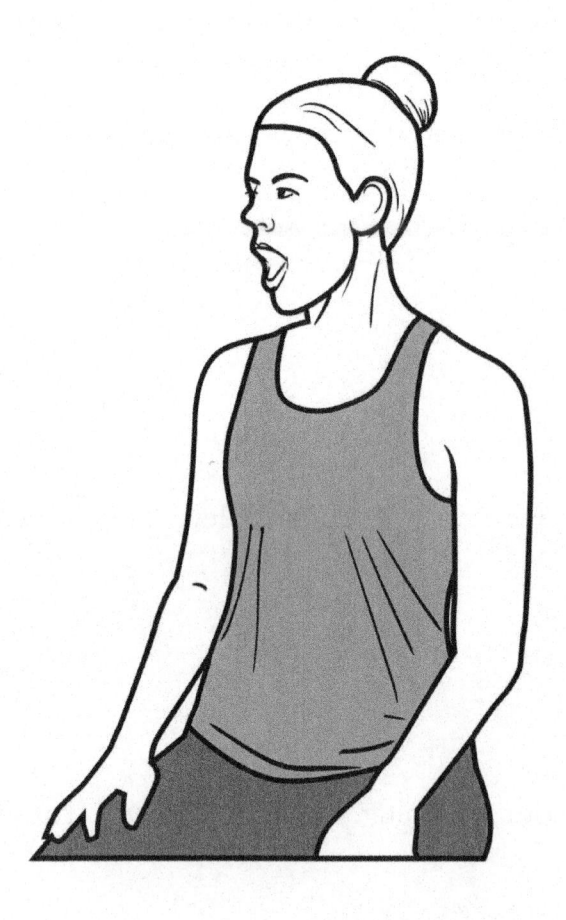

Level: Beginner

Another great way to stimulate your vagus nerve is through vocalization. Music is one of the best ways to connect with each other and ourselves. After all, some of the best albums were written from strong emotion, whether from heartbreak or anger. There is something to be said about vocalizing your feelings. But, as it turns out, you don't need to be a gifted singer to be able to benefit from vocalization.

Humming in particular tones has an incredible effect on our vagus nerve. These tones are quite similar to the ancient "aum" chanting you might be familiar with. You don't have to be particularly skilled or talented to be able to make this humming exercise work for you.

1. **Begin by taking a breath from deep in your abdomen.**

2. **On your exhale, make the "mmm" sound:** Really feel that vibration of the "mmm" sound.

3. **Do this as many times as is comfortable:** You want to get comfortable with it.

4. **Now, take another deep breath from your abdomen.**

5. **This time, on the exhale, drop your jaw and make an "ahh" sound:** You want your jaw to be loose, just dropping open as you make this sound. Don't force the exhale; let it come out evenly. Make the sound like there is a big apple in the back of your throat, stretching the throat.

6. **Repeat as many times as is comfortable:** Lengthen the exhale each time.

7. **Take another deep belly breath.**

8. **Now, make an "ooo" sound:** On your exhale, make a steady "ooo" sound.

9. **Bring them all together on your next exhale:** "Mmm–aaah–ooo–mm."

10. **Experiment with your exhale length and volume:** Get comfortable with it, and allow yourself to feel the relaxation being triggered through the vagus nerve.

Workbook Exercises

1. After humming, what sensations did you feel in your body?

2. What emotions did you feel?

Exercise 47: Gargling

One of the best things about stimulating the vagus nerve is the reduction in the stress and anxiety that we feel. But it's not the only benefit, of course. Every nonvoluntary system in the body benefits from vagus nerve stimulation. You might notice that you start to have an easier time with digestion. Or maybe your heart rate has begun to slow down. Whatever the case, practicing vagus nerve stimulation as part of your weekly, or even daily, routine will help you immensely in the long run.

Gargling is another simple way to use your throat to activate the vagus nerve. Remember, the vagus nerve comes down from our head all the way down to our large intestine. One of the benefits of its size is that there are multiple points in the body where you can work toward triggering the wanted response.

Gargling can also strengthen the vagus nerve. Believe it or not, we need to tone the vagus nerve a bit like a muscle to ensure that it is in a healthy condition. When you gargle, you are stimulating and "toning" it, making for a healthier overall nervous system. A healthier, more toned vagus nerve has been correlated with a higher chance of surviving cancer. This is because higher vagus nerve tone can actually slow the rate of tumor growth in some cases (Bullock, 2024). And gargling is such a simple way to help make that happen!

1. **Vigorously gargle warm water:** Do this one to two times a day for 30–60 seconds each time.

2. **Spit.**

3. **Add more sessions as needed:** If you are under more stress, feel free to add more gargling sessions.

Workbook Exercises

1. What did you feel after gargling?

2. Notice your breathing and describe the quality of it (e.g., deep, slow, full).

_____

_____

_____

Emotional Expression and Release

Emotions are a bit like nature. Like the changing of the seasons, they come and they go. They aren't a fixture. They are always ebbing and flowing along with circumstances, relationships, and change. We are capable of such strong and beautiful emotions as part of the human race, but unfortunately, society often conditions us to hide and even suppress our emotions. We're supposed to seem "strong" and "tough," and for many, that means stuffing sadness, anger, and grief down below the surface.

However, harboring emotions in secret is often our downfall. Emotions are energy in motion. So, what happens when we try to stifle an emotion? It gets stuck in the body. This can manifest as stomachaches, muscle tension, headaches, and more. The more we try to mask or stifle what we're feeling, the more stuck and tense we become.

So, then, what's the solution? Expressing that emotion! You want to find a way to get your emotions back out into the open. Whether verbally or through the body, expressing your emotions can have a significant impact on the mind–body connection. Healing from trauma and anxiety is impossible without allowing ourselves an emotional outlet of some kind.

Exercise 48: Twist and Growl

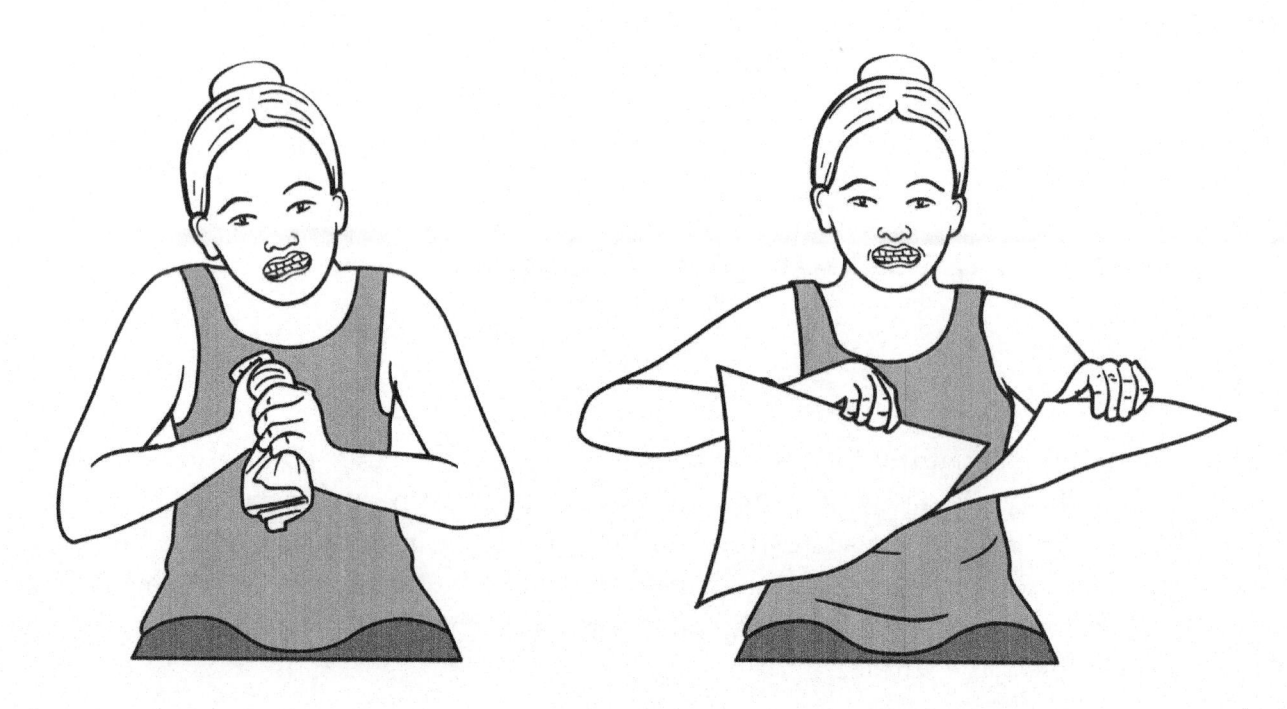

Level: Beginner

Every emotion serves its purpose. We have, over time, demonized certain emotions, but the fact is, they are all necessary if we are to be emotionally healthy. And denying those emotions is not what we want. There are no negative or positive emotions. They are all a beautiful part of being human, and they all tell us something about ourselves and the world around us.

Anger, for instance, is not negative. Rather, it is just a natural part of the human experience. When we feel the energy of anger begin to build in us, we need to express it in some way. The key is finding healthy and safe ways to express anger. Because, in the end, it takes more energy to suppress anger than it does to express it.

Let's take a look at the science of anger before heading into the next exercise. Anger, like fear, generates a stress response. Your heartbeat will get faster, your muscles will start to contract, and your body language will completely change. However, unlike with fear, you are more likely to choose confrontation over fleeing. Your body is literally preparing you for a physical conflict, whether or not you are planning on acting that out (Das, 2022).

While lashing out irrationally is bad for both your physical and mental health, keeping anger in can also be detrimental—because that energy has to go somewhere. And if you are denying it, you're likely to find yourself tensed up, wreaking havoc on the body *and* mind.

In this exercise, we will take a look at a way to express anger. Though we will be vocalizing it, we won't be using words. Sometimes, words fail us anyway. Let's take a look at how we can growl and twist out our anger.

1. **You will need a dish towel for this exercise:** However, you can also use a rag, washcloth, or any other medium-size piece of cloth.

2. **Grab a fistful of fabric with each hand on opposite ends of the cloth:** You want to make sure the fabric is folded up enough to give you that full feeling.

3. **Channel your anger through your arms and hands, into the dishtowel:** Give that dish towel one big twist. Bear down.

4. **Repeat.**

5. **Pause, take a moment, and tune in with your body:** What are you feeling physically and mentally?

6. **If needed, twist the dish towel again, vocalizing a growl as you do so.**

7. **Rest again, and have curiosity about your feelings again.**

8. **Feel free to use protective gloves, if that makes you feel safer in the exercise:** Alternatively, you might want to try ripping paper!

Workbook Exercises

1. What surprised you about doing the exercise, if anything?

2. What sensations did you feel in your body when doing this exercise? How about after?

Exercise 49: Laughter Yoga

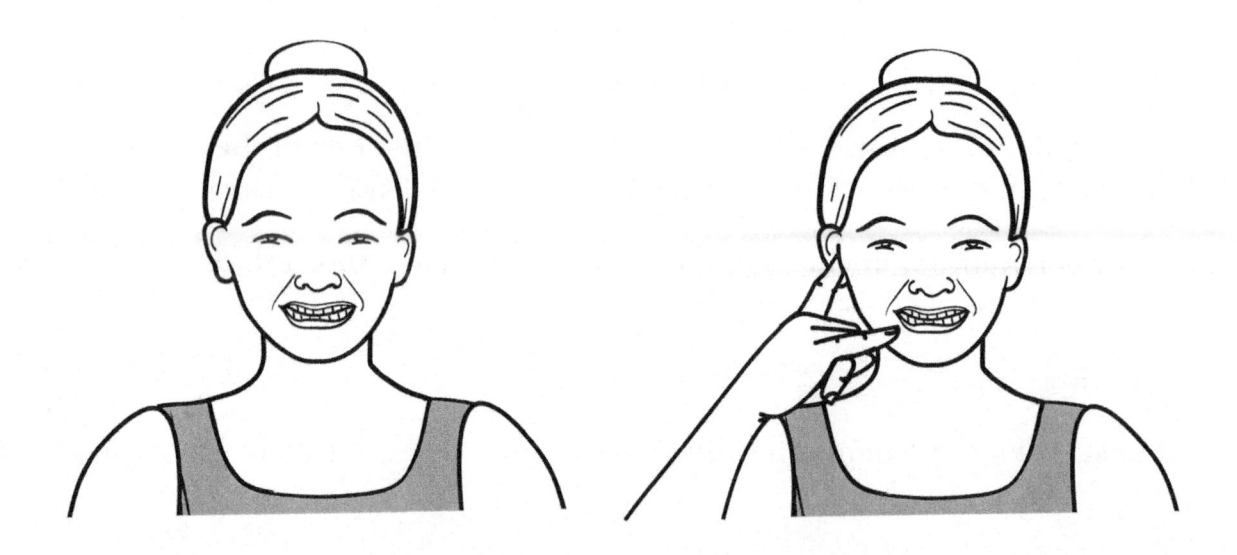

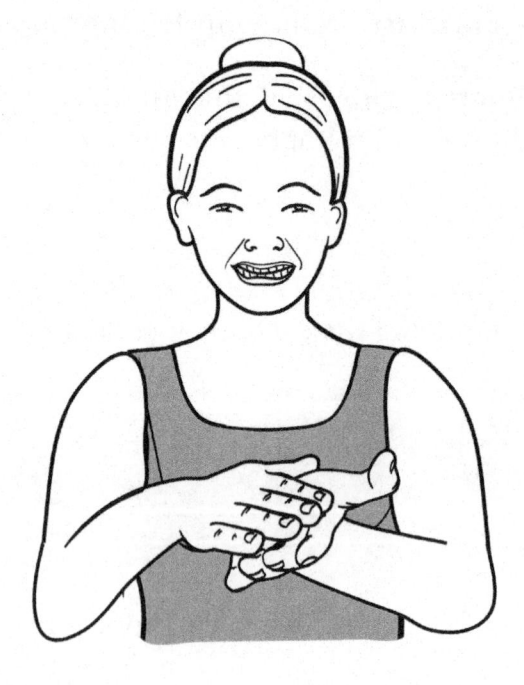

Level: Beginner

It isn't just feelings like anger that need to be expressed. Whether it's sadness or joy, all emotions have a place at the table and should be expressed in a healthy way.

This next exercise might be a little out of your comfort zone. Even if it feels a little awkward, silly, or uncomfortable, I give you permission to practice it anyway. Sometimes, we need something a little silly and awkward to shake us out of our rut. It gives us the chance to try something new and not take ourselves so seriously. Sometimes, there is laughter even in healing.

Have you ever laughed long and deep, and felt better afterward? Believe it or not, it's about a lot more than just the joy that made you laugh in the first place. Laughter itself can be incredibly beneficial. And it's not just emotional. We also get remarkable physiological benefits from the act, not the least of which is the drop in cortisol levels. But it can also positively impact blood pressure and lead to a decrease in depression scores (Louie et al., 2016).

And this refers to simulated laughter as well! For this exercise, we'll be pairing laughter with breathwork and some light yoga. Altogether, it makes for a great way to get anything out of your system, burn some energy, and allow your cortisol levels to drop.

1. **First, smile for a minute:** Really exaggerate it. Stretch it out. For that full moment, allow the smile to take up your full face.

2. **Now, hold your hand up to your face like it's a phone.**

3. **Laugh as you hold up that phone:** Again, do this for a full minute. Really lean into it.

4. **Pretend to wash your hands:** Now, laugh as you go through the motions of washing your hands.

5. **Remember:** You don't need to actually be laughing. As long as you are pretending to laugh, you are working the same muscles and taking in the same amount of oxygen. It still works.

Workbook Exercises

1. How did you feel doing the exercise (e.g., awkward, weird, funny)?

2. Did that initial feeling shift as you got deeper into the exercise? If so, how?

Exercise 50: Wiping the Table

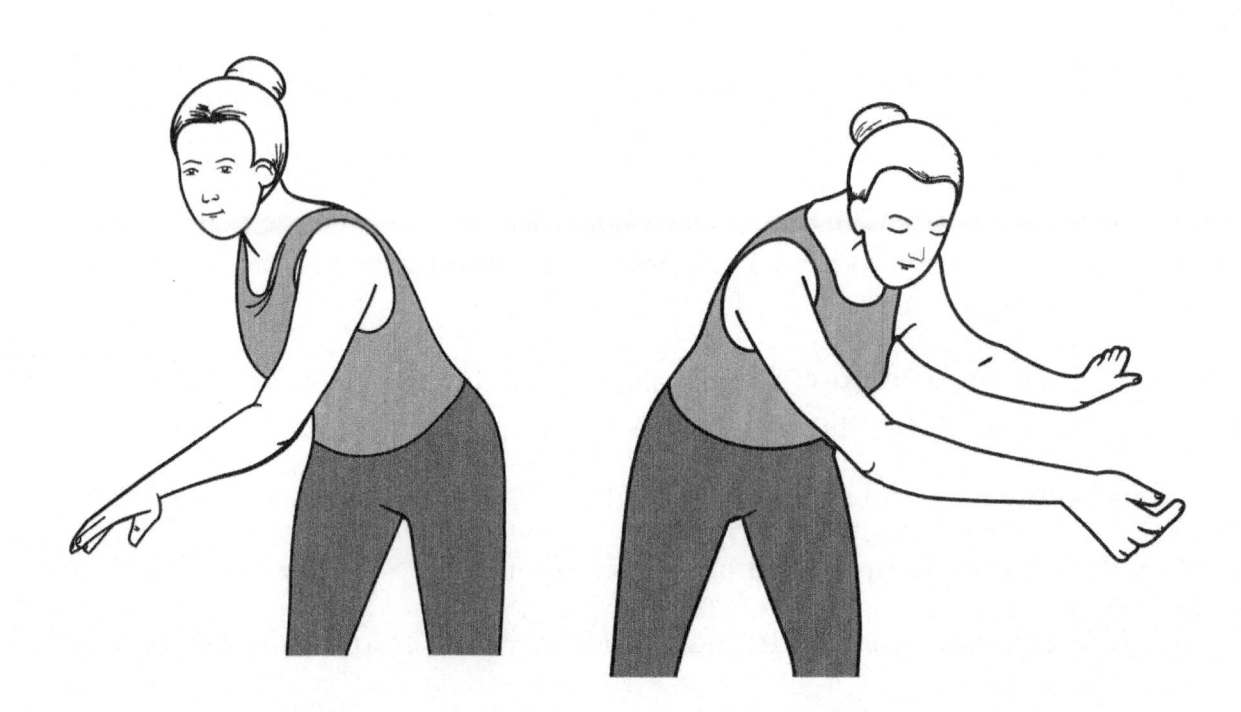

Sometimes, it works best to express emotions through our physical body. After all, we do that without even thinking sometimes. We wring our hands when we're nervous, or we laugh when we're feeling joyful. We might even run or jump up and down if we're excited. By expelling that energy in motion, we are releasing the emotions that might be stuck within our bodies.

We often hold our emotions in our fascia—the connective tissue that wraps around structures within the body—so we want to start there. In this exercise, we'll be "unsticking" emotions from the fascia through movement. Let's begin.

1. **Start by standing up:** Your feet should be a little wider than shoulder-width apart. Your arms should be loose at your sides.

2. **Now, make a dramatic wiping motion with your arms across your body:** Think of it like wiping down a table. You want to get everything off that table, so use big sweeping motions. It might help to bend your knees and lean forward.

3. **Imagine that what you are wiping away are the emotions you need to release:** If you are feeling anger, resentment, or frustration, let it flow out and get swept away by the wiping arm movement. Let your body flow.

4. **Check in with your body:** How do you feel? There is no right or wrong.

Workbook Exercises

1. What emotions wanted to be expressed while you did the exercise?

   _____

   _____

2. How were these emotions expressed through you (e.g., more vigorous movements, growling, yelling, crying, etc.)?

Exercise 51: Ecstatic Dancing

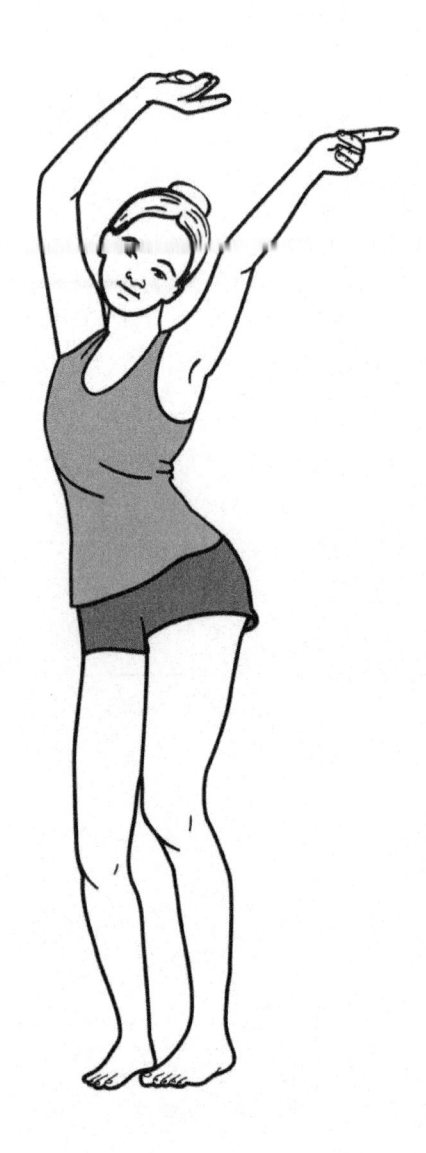

Dancing isn't just a workout for your body. Recent studies have found that participating in structured dance for a six-week period can have significant benefits for your cognitive and psychological well-being (Print & Blowes, 2024). Structured dance was not only equal to other types of exercise in this area, but at times *more* effective.

And you don't have to be particularly talented to feel the benefits. It isn't about skill level or ability. It's about the exercise itself. This next exercise is a lot of fun, but also a little different from some of our other exercises. I want you to know at the outset that there is no wrong way to participate. Listen to your body and modify the steps as necessary. Finally, music is a big part of this exercise. Turn on something that motivates you to dance! Have fun with it.

1. **Start by warming up your body:** Sway to the music, shifting from foot to foot in time with the music. Keep your arms loose, and move them at your sides as you sway and move.

2. **Now, try moving your feet:** Lift your feet when you're comfortable, alternating between them.

3. **Loosen up your shoulders as you begin to move your arms more.**

4. **Move your chest:** Again, loosely and freely, move your chest to the sides, continuing to move your arms.

5. **Move to expand and open your body:** You want to do big movements that open up your body language.

6. **Anything is okay as far as movement goes:** Just do what feels right.

7. **Start moving faster:** Let yourself feel ecstasy and excitement as you speed up your movements a bit.

8. **Don't hold your breath:** Make sure you are breathing freely and evenly.

9. **If your body is becoming hot, you are doing great!**

10. **Keep moving to the song, letting the energy flow inside:** The moves themselves are less important than how you are moving. Keep your body open and active.

11. **Speed up again:** Move your body more proactively, leaning into those feelings of ecstasy. Bounce around, wave your arms—just keep moving.

12. **Let the life force inside of you feel joy and ecstasy:** Let it feel free!

13. **Move every part of your body as you loosen up more:** There's no right or wrong; just keep moving! Keep the energy flowing.

14. **Feel the energy generating inside of you as you work it out of you:** Feelings of anxiety and sadness are leaving your body, being replaced with joy and lightness.

15. **Begin to slow down your movements:** Stay connected to your body, still feeling the energy flowing throughout you.

16. **Keep slowing down as you wind down the exercise until you find a comfortable place to stop:** Feel grateful for this moment, your body, and your life.

Workbook Exercises

1. What emotions came up for you as you danced in this exercise?

2. How did your body feel after the exercise?

Part 3: 28-Day Plan

Feel free to use this 28-day plan to start your somatic journey! Having a plan when starting out is often beneficial, and this one can be done in as little as seven minutes a day. Give these exercises a try for the next 28 days and feel your nervous system begin to reset and heal.

Day 1: Body Scan (5 min) and Squeeze Hug (2 min)

Day 2: Monkey Stance (5 min) and Supportive Touch (5 min)

Day 3: Pursed-Lip Breathing (3 min) and Hand Reflexology (10 min)

Day 4: Gargling (2 min) and Release Neck and Shoulder Tension (10 min)

Day 5: Ecstatic Dancing (5 min), Squeeze Hug (3 min), and Softening the Gaze (2 min)

Day 6: Twist and Growl (5 min) and Opening (Qigong) (5 min)

Day 7: Bilateral Stimulation (10 min) and Humming (3 min)

Day 8: 4–5–6 Breathing (3 min) and Release Psoas (5 min)

Day 9: Brain Tapping (5 min) and Lifting the Ball (Qigong) (10 min)

Day 10: Laughing Yoga (5 min) and Tuning Into the Senses (5 min)

Day 11: Body Tapping (Qigong) (5 min) and Lessening Effort (5 min)

Day 12: Whispered "Ah" (Rediscovering Your Voice) (2 minutes), Butterfly Hug (5 min), and Body Scan (5 min)

Day 13: Softening the Gaze (2 min) and Wiping the Table (5 min)

Day 14: Double Inhale Technique (3 min), Protective Force Fields (5 min), and Gargling (1 min)

Day 15: Lying-Down Work (10 min) and Understanding Misuse vs. Proper Use (5 min)

Day 16: Cupping the Eyes (5 min), Shaking (Qigong) (5 min), and Diaphragmatic Breathing (2 min)

Day 17: Retraining the Neck and Shoulders (10 min), Lizard Walk (3 min), and Cupping the Eyes (2 min)

Day 18: Brain Tapping (5 min) and Release Psoas (7 min)

Day 19: Frolicking in Water (Qigong) (10 min) and Tuning Into the Senses (5 min)

Day 20: Emotional Freedom Technique (EFT) (5 min), Snap–Snap–Clap Rhythm (2 min), and 4–5–6 Breathing (3 min)

Day 21: Lifting the Ball (Qigong) (10 min), Ear Pull (2 min), and Whispered "Ah" (Rediscovering Your Voice) (3 min)

Day 22: Eye Movement Routine (Qigong) (5 minute) and Salamander Exercise (5 min)

Day 23: Swaying Bamboo (Qigong) (5 min) and Standing in Your Power (3 min)

Day 24: Tree Grounding Visualization (5 min), Ecstatic Dancing (5 min), and Three-Dimensional Breathing (3 min)

Day 25: Slight Chest Compressions (5 min) and Voo Breathing (3 min)

Day 26: 4–5–6 Breathing (3 min), Release Stomach Tension (5 min), and Monkey Stance (5 min)

Day 27: Diaphragmatic Breathing (3 min) and Progressive Muscle Relaxation (5 min)

Day 28: Three-Dimensional Breathing (3 min), Laughing Yoga (10 min), and Cupping the Eyes (2 min)

Conclusion

This journey through somatic exercises is a profound exploration of the mind–body connection. As you practice, you will learn to depend on these transformative tools for enhancing self-awareness, emotional regulation, and physical well-being. As we've discussed throughout the book, it is important to tune in and listen to your body. Somatic practices invite us to recognize our bodies as sources of wisdom rather than just vessels for our thoughts and emotions. By engaging in these exercises, we are releasing stored tension and trauma, but we're also cultivating a deeper sense of presence in our daily lives.

The benefits of somatic exercises extend far beyond the physical realm. Rather, they encourage us to reconnect with our bodily rhythms and instincts. In this, we find grounding and safety. Our world often prioritizes the cognitive over the corporeal, but somatic practices remind us to return to the valuable insights of our bodies.

As you embark on this journey of somatic practice, remember—this journey doesn't need to be linear. In fact, it is a deeply personal endeavor and should be taken at your own pace. There is no right or wrong way to listen to and engage with your body. Each of these practices is an opportunity to explore, to feel, and to learn. Ensure you are treating yourself with compassion and patience as you navigate forward.

Ultimately, somatic exercises serve as an invitation to reclaim our bodies. They are an integral part of our identity, and by embracing this holistic approach, we cultivate a more vibrant, authentic existence. I hope that you have found these exercises helpful, and that you can integrate them into your wellness journey. I wish you the best of luck!

Thank you so much for making it to the end!

I'm truly grateful you chose to read my book.

Among the dozens of other books you could have picked, you made the decision to take this journey with me, so a heartfelt THANK YOU for making it this far.

As we part ways (for now), I want to ask you for a small favor:

If you have 60 seconds, could you share your honest review on Amazon? Posting a review is the easiest way to support the work of independent authors like myself. I always love hearing how this powerful work impacts your life!

Easy steps to leave your feedback:

1. Open the camera app on your mobile or tablet device.

2. Point your device at the QR code below

3. The review page will show up in your web browser

References

Ali, M. M. (2022, May 24). *The science of visualization: Can imagining your goals make you more likely to accomplish them?* Neurovine. https://www.neurovine.ai/blog/the-science-of-visualization-can-imagining-your-goals-make-you-more-likely-to-accomplish-them

Ally, C. (2020, February 11). *Trauma care: "Voo" breathing.* Flourish Counseling Co. https://flourishcounseling.co/trauma-care-voo-breathing/

Bailey, E. (2021, May 7). *Caregiver burnout prevention: How body tapping helps increase your energy.* Elizabeth Bailey. https://elizabethbaileybooks.com/caregiver-burnout-prevention-body-tapping-energy-snacks/

Beer, J. (2024, August 6). *EFT tapping: The psychology behind tapping therapy.* PositivePsychology.com. https://positivepsychology.com/eft-tapping/

Braunsdorf, A. (2023, August 11). *A complete guide to bilateral stimulation.* Balance. https://balanceapp.com/blog/bilateral-stimulation

Bullock, B. G. (2024, April 1). *Vagus nerve activity may impact cancer prognosis.* YogaUOnline.com. https://yogauonline.com/yoga-and-healthy-aging/yoga-for-cancer/vagus-nerve-activity-may-impact-cancer-prognosis/

Cleveland Clinic. (n.d.-a). *Diaphragmatic breathing.* https://my.clevelandclinic.org/health/articles/9445-diaphragmatic-breathing

Cleveland Clinic. (n.d.-b). *Mouth breathing.* https://my.clevelandclinic.org/health/diseases/22734-mouth-breathing

Cleveland Clinic. (n.d.-c). *Pursed lip breathing.* https://my.clevelandclinic.org/health/treatments/9443-pursed-lip-breathing

Cleveland Clinic. (2023, February 3). *Body scan meditation for beginners: How to make the mind/body connection.* https://health.clevelandclinic.org/body-scan-meditation

Cronkleton, E. (2018, February 26). *Hand reflexology: How to cure anxiety, headaches, and constipation.* Healthline. https://www.healthline.com/health/hand-reflexology

Das, J. (2022, September 8). *Science of emotions: Understanding anger.* The Franklin Institute. https://fi.edu/en/blog/science-emotions-understanding-anger

Dooley, T. (2020, November 13). *TMJ pain relief: At-home exercise for your jaw.* Cedar Village Dentistry. https://cedarvillagedentistry.com/tmj-relief-at-home-exercises/

Farrell, A. (n.d.). *The whispered ah!* Alexander Technique London & Online. https://www.alexander-technique.london/articles/defining-the-alexander-technique/the-whispered-ah/

Filipiak, M. (n.d.). *Try the butterfly hug to help with PTSD symptoms.* Counseling Connections. https://www.counselingconnectionsnm.com/blog/try-the-butterfly-hug-to-help-with-ptsd-symptoms

Fletcher, J. (2019, February 12). *4-7-8 breathing: How it works, benefits, and uses.* Www.medicalnewstoday.com. https://www.medicalnewstoday.com/articles/324417

Frankl, V. (n.d.) *Viktor Frankl quotes.* Goodreads. https://www.goodreads.com/author/quotes/2782.Viktor_E_Frankl

Haden, J. (2023, January 27). *Stanford neuroscientist: This 5-second breathing technique is the fastest way to reduce anxiety and stress.* Inc. https://www.inc.com/jeff-haden/stanford-neuroscientist-this-5-second-breathing-technique-is-fastest-way-to-reduce-anxiety-stress.html

Hanna, T. (n.d.) *Thomas Hanna quotes.* A-Z Quotes. https://www.azquotes.com/author/56542-Thomas_Hanna

Harvard Health Publishing. (2023, September 29). *Past trauma may haunt your future health.* https://www.health.harvard.edu/diseases-and-conditions/past-trauma-may-haunt-your-future-health

Hilal, A., Bazarah, M., & Kapoula, Z. (2022). Benefits of implementing eye-movement training in the rehabilitation of patients with age-related macular degeneration: A review. *Brain Sciences, 12*(1), 36. https://doi.org/10.3390/brainsci12010036

How panoramic vision can reduce your stress and anxiety. (2022, August 8). Sandvi Studio. https://sandvistudio.com/blogs/news/panoramic-vision-destress-and-improve-posture

How posture affects neurological and cognitive function. (2024, April 23). BackEmbrace. https://backembrace.com/blogs/articles/how-posture-affects-neurological-and-cognitive-function

HYNS Team. (2023, December 18). *43 techniques to activate your parasympathetic nervous system and lower stress.* Heal Your Nervous System. https://healyournervoussystem.com/45-techniques-to-activate-your-parasympathetic-nervous-system-and-lower-stress/

Jagim, A. (2020, June 8). *The importance of movement.* Mayo Health Clinic System. https://www.mayoclinichealthsystem.org/hometown-health/featured-topic/the-importance-of-movement

Jahnke, R., Larkey, L., Rogers, C., Etnier, J., & Lin, F. (2010). A comprehensive review of health benefits of qigong and tai chi. *American Journal of Health Promotion*, *24*(6), e1–e25. https://doi.org/10.4278/ajhp.081013-LIT-248

König, N., Steber, S., Seebacher, J., von Prittwitz, Q., Bliem, H. R., & Rossi, S. (2019). How therapeutic tapping can alter neural correlates of emotional prosody processing in anxiety. *Brain Sciences*, *9*(8), 206. https://doi.org/10.3390/brainsci9080206

Loncar, T. (2021, June 8). *A decade of power posing: Where do we stand?* The British Psychological Society. https://www.bps.org.uk/psychologist/decade-power-posing-where-do-we-stand

Louie, D., Brook, K., & Frates, E. (2016). The laughter prescription. *American Journal of Lifestyle Medicine*, *10*(4), 262–267. https://doi.org/10.1177/1559827614550279

Mayo Clinic Staff. (2023, April 18). *Vagus nerve stimulation*. Mayo Clinic. https://www.mayoclinic.org/tests-procedures/vagus-nerve-stimulation/about/pac-20384565

Mazzei, R. (n.d.). *How bilateral stimulation can help you feel better*. Evolutions Behavioral Health Services. https://www.evolutionsbh.com/articles/how-bilateral-stimulation-can-help-you-feel-better/

Murnan, A. (2023, August 21). *Can emotions be trapped in the body? What to know*. Medical News Today. https://www.medicalnewstoday.com/articles/emotions-trapped-in-the-body

National Center for Complementary and Integrative Health. (2022, February). *Qigong: What you need to know*. https://nccih.nih.gov/health/qigong-what-you-need-to-know

Nitka, D. (2017, May 16). *The importance of setting boundaries*. Connecte Psychology. https://connectepsychology.com/en/2017/05/16/the-importance-of-setting-boundaries/

Ortego, G., Villafañe, J. H., Doménech-García, V., Berjano, P., Bertozzi, L., & Herrero, P. (2016). Is there a relationship between psychological stress or anxiety and chronic nonspecific neck-arm pain in adults? A systematic review and meta-analysis. *Journal of Psychosomatic Research*, *90*, 70–81. https://doi.org/10.1016/j.jpsychores.2016.09.006

Paturel, A. (2024, March 21). *Bolster your brain by stimulating the vagus nerve*. Cedars-Sinai. https://www.cedars-sinai.org/blog/stimulating-the-vagus-nerve.html

Print, K., & Blowes, M. (2024, February 12). *Dancing may be better than other exercise for improving mental health*. The University of Sydney. https://www.sydney.edu.au/news-opinion/news/2024/02/12/dancing-may-be-better-than-other-exercise-for-improving-mental-h.html

Rejeh, N., Tadrisi, S. D., Yazdani, S., Saatchi, K., & Vaismoradi, M. (2020). The effect of hand reflexology massage on pain and fatigue in patients after coronary angiography: A randomized controlled clinical trial. *Nursing Research and Practice, 2020*, 8386167. https://doi.org/10.1155/2020/8386167

Schwede, M. (2024, February 17). *The captivating benefits of rocking while sleeping: How Swing2Sleep is based on scientific findings.* Swing2Sleep.com. https://www.swing2sleep.com/blogs/news/the-captivating-benefits-of-rocking-while-sleeping-how-swing2sleep-is-based-on-scientific-findings

Selhub, E. (2015, November 23). *The Alexander technique can help you (literally) unwind.* Harvard Health Publishing. https://www.health.harvard.edu/blog/the-alexander-technique-can-help-you-literally-unwind-201511238652

Siccardi, M. A., Tariq, M. A., & Valle, C. (2020). *Anatomy, bony pelvis and lower limb: Psoas major.* StatPearls Publishing. https://www.ncbi.nlm.nih.gov/books/NBK535418/

Tanasugarn, A. (2022, November 5). *The health risks of a dysregulated nervous system.* Psychology Today. https://www.psychologytoday.com/us/blog/understanding-ptsd/202211/the-health-risks-dysregulated-nervous-system

Toner, J. (n.d.). *Pandiculation - the benefits of stretching like a cat.* Ekhart Yoga. https://www.ekhartyoga.com/articles/practice/pandiculation-the-benefits-of-stretching-like-a-cat

Tomlinson, C. (2021, October 1). *4 easy exercises for the eyes.* Yoga Journal. https://www.yogajournal.com/lifestyle/health/2020-vision-quest/

Toussaint, L., Nguyen, Q. A., Roettger, C., Dixon, K., Offenbächer, M., Kohls, N., Hirsch, J., & Sirois, F. (2021). Effectiveness of progressive muscle relaxation, deep breathing, and guided imagery in promoting psychological and physiological states of relaxation. *Evidence-Based Complementary and Alternative Medicine, 2021*, 5924040. https://doi.org/10.1155/2021/5924040

Tsong, N. (2023, October 7). This intense lizard-crawl workout will bring you to your knees. *The Seattle Times.* https://seattletimes.com/pacific-nw-magazine/this-intense-lizard-crawl-workout-will-bring-you-to-your-knees/

Vinall, M. (2021, March 5). *Can shaking your body help heal stress and trauma? Some experts say yes.* Healthline. https://www.healthline.com/health/mental-health/can-shaking-your-body-heal-stress-and-trauma

Vivos. (2022, December 16). *Improper breathing and its negative effects on your health.* https://vivos.com/improper-breathing-and-its-negative-effects-on-your-health/

Warren, S. (2022, April 21). *What is pandiculation?* Somatic Movement Center. https://somaticmovementcenter.com/pandiculation-what-is-pandiculation/

World Health Organization. (2024, May 27). *Post-traumatic stress disorder.* https://www.who.int/news-room/fact-sheets/detail/post-traumatic-stress-disorder

Printed in Great Britain
by Amazon